TRAUMA: CODE RED

COMPANION TO THE RCSEng DEFINITIVE
SURGICAL TRAUMA SKILLS COURSE

TRAUMA: CODE RED

COMPANION TO THE RCSEng DEFINITIVE SURGICAL TRAUMA SKILLS COURSE

Edited by

Mansoor Khan, MBBS PhD FRCS FEBS FACS AKC
Surgeon Commander Royal Navy
Consultant Trauma and Military Surgeon
St Mary's Hospital Major Trauma Centre
London, United Kingdom

Morgan McMonagle, MB BCh BAO MD FRCSI FACS
Consultant General
and
Trauma and Vascular Surgeon
St Mary's Hospital Major Trauma Centre
London, United Kingdom
and The South/South West Hospital Group, Ireland

with

David M. Nott, OBE DSc MD FRCS DMCC
Professor of Conflict Surgery, Imperial College London
and
Consultant Vascular and Trauma Surgeon
St Mary's Hospital Major Trauma Centre
London, United Kingdom

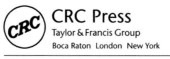
CRC Press
Taylor & Francis Group
Boca Raton London New York

CRC Press is an imprint of the
Taylor & Francis Group, an **informa** business

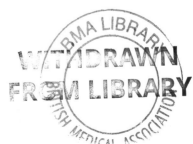

This book is dedicated to all those, especially the victims and their families, affected by the mass terrorist atrocities that have occurred on UK soil in the past two decades, in particular the London bombings of 7th July 2005, the Westminster Bridge attack of 22nd March 2017, the Manchester Arena bombing of 22nd May 2017 and the London Bridge attack of 3rd June 2017. We must also give special mention to the dedicated first responders and pre-hospital care providers (bystanders, fire service, police and ambulance crew) and hospital staff (clinical, nursing and ancillary) whose enduring spirit never fails to rise to meet all challenges at any time, well above and beyond the call of duty. It is this profound devotion and *esprit de corps* that keeps a health service and society at large alive during times of crisis.

'If you're going through hell, keep going'

—Winston Churchill

Mansoor Khan
Morgan McMonagle
David M. Nott

Contents

Foreword by David Feliciano, MD

While general surgery has become increasingly fragmented into subspecialties, trauma remains the one area in which a broad-based knowledge of anatomy, evaluation, principles of non-operative management and operative skills is mandatory. Working in such a surgical field poses a unique problem for practising surgeons, fellows, residents and medical students – i.e. how best to learn and then maintain the knowledge and skills necessary to care appropriately for every injured patient arriving in the trauma room.

The Definitive Surgical Trauma Care (DSTC) course evolved from the 'Guidelines for Essential Trauma Care' first developed by the International Association for the Surgery of Trauma and Surgical Intensive Care/International Society of Surgery and published by the World Health Organization in 2004. The goal of this document was to promote 'inexpensive improvements in facility-based trauma care', recognising the significant disparities in trauma care between 'high-income countries' versus 'middle- and low-income countries'. The Definitive Surgical Trauma Skills course was subsequently developed by the Royal College of Surgeons of England with the Royal Defence Medical College and the Uniformed University of the Health Sciences in Bethesda, Maryland, USA.

The Definitive Surgical Trauma Skills Course is of great value as a one-stop source for learning how to perform procedures and operations in all systems of the body. *Trauma: Code Red*, this new text by Mansoor Khan and Morgan McMonagle from St Mary's Hospital Major Trauma Center in London, United Kingdom, can stand alone as a consolidated textbook of trauma or be used as a companion to the RCSEng Definitive Surgical Trauma Skills Course. The content is unique in that, following the introductory chapters on damage control and ballistics, every other chapter is directed at definitive and damage control approaches to clinical management. These include management of the airway, injuries to the chest, abdomen, and pelvis, vascular injuries and fasciotomy of the extremities, and, finally, a comprehensive review of the emerging role of resuscitative endovascular balloon occlusion of the aorta (REBOA) in truncal trauma.

Each chapter, written by recognised authorities in the field of trauma, contains an introductory outline, operative photographs complemented by instructional line drawings, comprehensive line drawings describing techniques of exposure, pertinent tables and a reading list. The reader will be rewarded with a highly practical textbook/atlas of management that can be referred to in the trauma room or even in the operating room.

As trauma systems continue to improve around the world, there are more patients than ever with life- and/or limb-threatening injuries arriving at trauma centres. Many of these patients died in the field or during transit in the past. The practical skills highlighted in this new textbook will unequivocally save lives by educating trauma surgeons in appropriate and rapid resuscitation and operative management.

David V. Feliciano, MD

Clinical Professor of Surgery, University of Maryland School of Medicine
Attending Surgeon, Shock Trauma Center/Department of Surgery
University of Maryland Medical Center
22 South Greene Street, S4D07
Baltimore, MD 21201-1595

The Emergency Repair Specialist's Handbook, Volume 1

The term *damage control* comes from the United States Navy's system of rapidly deploying measures to maintain or restore a ship's integrity when damaged, to allow it a safe exit from hostile environments, and to definitively repair damages, so that it might 'live to fight another day.' The individuals responsible for delivering damage control aboard such vessels are called damage controlmen and are described within their manuals as *emergency repair specialists* (picture below). Navy damage controlmen provide efforts related to damage control, ship stability, and more. As well, they instruct other naval personnel in the methods of damage control and in the repair of damage control equipment and systems. The damage control manuals are exhaustive as is the training of these individuals.

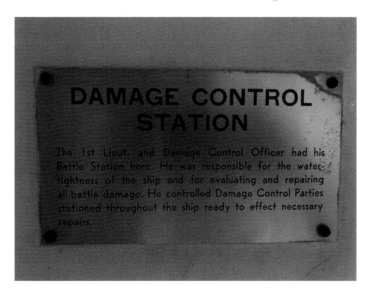

The current generation of surgeons, while never knowing a time without damage control, has only had this experience and knowledge passed down, so to speak, as an oral history from their faculty surgeons. The trainee may have previously picked up knowledge from the occasional book chapter on the subject. With the recent adoption and promotion of courses such as DSTS, surgical trainees and practicing surgeons can now receive hands-on experience in damage control philosophy and techniques from masters and experts in the field. However, until now, there has never been a true book to codify these principles and put into writing these techniques and the reason behind them, further supplementing the amazing education and experience these courses have passed along.

Trauma: Code Red takes the learner from underlying philosophy of damage control to the various unique maneuvers and master-level management techniques that one receives during these courses. Khan and McMonagle have finally made this knowledge available to the learner to take with them, keeping the wisdom, pearls, and consultant advice at but arms length. The book begins, appropriately, with lessons on the philosophy of damage control, delivered by authors from Penn, who coined the term and expanded and matured the concept over the last several decades. The authors then delve into the violent mechanisms that lead the severely injured patients to our doorsteps, going farther than the usual $KE = 1/2MV^2$. By doing so, the authors bring critical perspective to the devices responsible for the damage and wisdom as to their likely impact on the patient's tissues. Not missing a beat, the book then proceeds through the surgical ABCs of trauma, with subsequent chapters on emergency airway, chest injures, and vascular trauma. As with the course itself, the book's coverage of the surgical airway simultaneously maintains the learner's appropriate 'sphincter tone' while helping to guide them confidently and competently through what it is often a chaotic (and almost always unplanned) situation. The book then transitions from life to limb scenarios with ample and expert-level discussion and descriptions of pelvic and extremity trauma, along with the concomitant procedures to save both life and limb. Next, the editors have included THE chapter that is most critical to such a discussion, but is most often omitted as assumed knowledge and comfort: Damage Control Laparotomy. The chapter guides (and reminds) the learner through appropriate positioning, the 'stem-to-stern' incision, exposures to expedite control of bleeding, and the techniques to best secure hemostasis by injury and body region. The book then wraps up with a fantastic yet concise instruction on approaching individual abdominal injuries as well as a discussion of the future of damage control care, including a thoughtful inclusion of REBOA by Morrison and colleagues.

Along with the fantastic courses offered by the RCS Eng and others, this book will help to provide confidence and competence in providing the initial care of these patients. It may also help to inspire a generation of trainees to follow the lead of many of the authors of *Trauma: Code Red* into the field of trauma surgery. If we are lucky, they might even end up restoring the field to 'Big T' status, training them to care for any injury, head to toe, and help them achieve full *Emergency Repair Specialist* status.

Bryan A. Cotton, MD, MPH

John B Holmes Professor of Clinical Sciences
Director, Surgical Critical Care, Acute Care Surgery and Trauma Fellowships
Department of Surgery and The Center for Translational Injury Research
McGovern Medical School at The University of Texas Health Science Center at Houston
Assistant Director, Shock-Trauma ICU
Red Duke Trauma Institute at Memorial Hermann Hospital

Preface

Trauma surgery is the last great frontier of general surgery! Only a well-trained and experienced trauma surgeon will venture into any injured territory (neck, chest, abdomen, pelvis and limbs) no matter what the danger (massive haemorrhage). It is often difficult to define what is meant by the description 'experienced'. We prefer to describe the *experienced surgeon* as *one who is comfortable managing an uncomfortable situation!* This is certainly a requirement in effectively managing the polytrauma patient, presenting in shock with non-compressible torso haemorrhage, in addition to potential bleeding in the abdomen and pelvis simultaneously. The patient rapidly begins to decompensate. What do I do? Which cavity needs exploration first? How do I gain rapid haemorrhage control after opening and before patient demise? What are the surgical priorities? Is a trauma bay thoracotomy indicated? Unfortunately, the correct answers to these questions has been distorted by numerous other trauma dicta over the past 30 years, mandating vigorous fluid resuscitation before surgery and delaying decision making pending the patient response. In addition, although non-operative management of many injuries is well-described and accepted, we feel this pendulum has swung too far in the wrong direction. Many acute care surgeons now fail to recognise the very important cohort of patients that are unsuitable for non-operative management and who are in addition, uncomfortable with open surgery for trauma. What if that surgeon is you?

Unfortunately, we are seeing an increasing number of trauma patients year upon year as a result of accidents and intentional harm. In addition, the last decade has seen an increase in terrorist activity globally with a simultaneous increase in complex casualties. Injuries which historically were confined to the battlefield are now seen frequently in the civilian environment.

The bulk of severe injuries are now concentrated within major trauma centres (MTCs). Trauma experience is now more confined to such specialist centres, but the smaller trauma units continue to play a very important role in the network, especially regarding decision-making; those in need of transfer to the MTC, those in need of acute damage control prior to transportation or those injuries that may be managed locally.

It is widely recognised that over 50% of patients that die in the first 4 hours following major trauma die either directly from haemorrhage or haemorrhage is a major contributing factor in their death. This may be confounded by the demise of the true 'general surgeon' and/or a lack of experience in operative surgery and complex decision-making for trauma. Subspecialisation has led to focused training within individual specialties, with limited exposure to other areas of surgical practice, including emergency general surgery and especially trauma. Therefore, today's surgeons are less comfortable in dealing with other injured regions of the body or extremes of physiology that they do not encounter on a regular basis.

During our training and subsequent surgical practice, we have had the privilege of working with some truly remarkable surgeons and patients, in particular at world-class trauma facilities including Penn Trauma at the Hospital of the University of Pennsylvania (Philadelphia, United States); the Shock Trauma Center at the University of Maryland, Medical Center in Baltimore (Maryland, United States); and the Role 3 Hospital at Camp Bastion, Afghanistan. These individuals and facilities have allowed us to hone and direct our clinical skills, knowledge and surgical acumen to enable better care for the severely injured. The true reward is being able to give back to the surgical fraternity in terms of education all that we have learnt in the past two decades.

This book is both a stand-alone textbook and is the companion book to the internationally acclaimed Royal College of Surgeons of England 'Definitive Surgical Trauma Skills' course. We aim to simplify complex decision-making for the trauma patient and provide a simple didactic approach. It is a damage control book and a damage control course. It is a book and course on how to manage post-traumatic exsanguinating haemorrhage. Although difficult to define objectively, exsanguination is more of a recognition than a definition; *exsanguinating haemorrhage is the bleeding patient at risk of losing their entire blood volume within minutes.* Once recognised, the surgeon must now decide on the most compelling site of exsanguination. The book and course aim to facilitate the recognition of this in addition to enhanced complex decision-making surrounding it, especially in the search for and surgical management of the most compelling bleeding source.

Both the book and course aim to give the reader insights from world-class experts on damage control based on decades of experience, exposure and training. Alongside expert but simplified illustrations, the text aims to provide a step-by-step guide on what to do when the surgeon (perhaps less familiar with the trauma environment) is feeling uncomfortable in an uncomfortable situation. We hope that this book, in addition to the the damage control course, will enable the surgeon on trauma call to begin to feel more familiar and less uncomfortable, perhaps even comfortable when dealing with the time-critical, severely injured patient, perhaps turning a potential horror story into a feel-good experience.

We all hope that no one gets injured. However, if you are involved in treating the severely injured, we truly believe that this text will provide invaluable assistance into the management of major trauma patients.

Surgeons leave this course armed with new techniques – given that 'general' surgeons are rare beings, and new strategies and tactics for dealing with the single, most common post-trauma cause of death: non-compressible haemorrhage. This course that has undoubtedly improved (significantly) the survival rate in the UK for victims of severe torso trauma. The value of the DSTS course, superseded by the Military Operational Surgical Training (MOST) Course and Surgical Training for the Austere Environments (STAE) courses, is self-evident, when the massive improvement in survivors wounded in Iraq and Afghanistan, is noted.

The late Peter Roberts, CBE SM MS FRCS
Professor Emeritus of Military Surgery
Royal College of Surgeons of England

Mansoor Khan

Morgan McMonagle

Editors

Mansoor Khan, MBBS (Lond), PhD, FRCS (GenSurg), FEBS (GenSurg), FACS, AKC, is a Consultant Trauma Surgeon at the North West London Major Trauma Centre based at St Mary's Hospital, Paddington as well as a Surgeon Commander in the Royal Navy. After graduation from King's College London in 2000, he undertook his House Officer training in Plymouth and Portsmouth, followed by three years of military posts. In November 2001 he graduated from Britannia Royal Naval College in Dartmouth and was deployed in the Northern Arabian Gulf on military operations upon completion. The remainder of his general duties saw deployments in the Baltic and North Sea on NATO's Immediate Reaction Force of Minehunters, the 2003 Gulf War and counter narcotics deployment in the Caribbean.

Upon completion of three years of military general duties, he commenced surgical training completing his rotations in Peterborough, Birmingham and South Yorkshire. After having successfully obtained his FRCS in General Surgery in 2010, he was subsequently deployed on tour at Camp Bastion in Afghanistan, followed by a 1-year Trauma Critical Care Fellowship at the world-renowned R Adams Cowley Shock-Trauma Center in Baltimore, Maryland, USA. He was appointed as consultant general surgeon in the Defence Medical Services of the United Kingdom, and subsequently was awarded Fellowship of the European Board of Surgery and Fellowship of the American College of Surgeons. Since appointment as a Consultant Trauma Surgeon he has undertaken multiple operational tours in addition to lead clinician for the military team awarded the Military Civilian Health Partnership Award, 2014 for Team of the Year. He is a member of the American Association for the Surgery of Trauma.

The current military positions include; Consultant Advisor in General Surgery to the Medical Director, General Royal Navy and Senior Lecturer in Military Surgery at the Royal Centre for Defence Medicine. Civilian positions include Honorary Senior Lecturer at Imperial College London, National Institute for Health Research (NIHR) academic, editor/associate editor and reviewer for multiple journals, undergraduate and postgraduate examiner, Co-Director of the Definitive Surgical Trauma Skills course at the Royal College of Surgeons of England as well as faculty on multiple international surgical training courses. He is keen on research and has published extensively with over 170 publications, book chapters and conference papers.

His interests include primary injury prevention research, blast mitigation strategies, haemorrhage control, trauma education, physiological monitoring and studying the gut microbiome in relation to trauma and hypoperfusion.

Morgan McMonagle, MB, BCh, BAO (Hons), MD, FRCSI, FACS is a consultant trauma surgeon in the North West London Trauma Network based at St Mary's Hospital, London and a general and vascular surgeon with the South/South West Hospital Group in Ireland. After graduating from University College Dublin (UCD) with honours in 1997, he undertook basic surgical training at the Royal College of Surgeons in Ireland (RCSI) hospital group after which he gained further trauma surgery experience at Westmead Hospital, Sydney, Australia. Following this he gained extensive experience working in prehospital care and aeromedical retrieval with Careflight™ and Careflight™ International, Australia and later with MAGPAS air ambulance in the United Kingdom. He completed higher surgical training with the West Midlands surgical training programme, UK followed by a Vascular & Endovascular Fellowship at the Royal Brisbane & Women's hospital, Brisbane, Australia. He then undertook additional fellowship training in trauma, emergency surgery and surgical critical care at the world renowned and prestigious trauma programme Penn-Trauma at the Hospital of the University of Pennsylvania, USA, after which he was awarded fellowship of the American College of Surgeons (FACS). As well as being faculty on the NECPOD report Trauma: who cares? (2007), which was instrumental in the development of the UK trauma network, he was the first trauma surgeon appointed at Imperial Healthcare as part of the new London Trauma Network. He was also faculty member on the steering group advising on the document *A Trauma System for Ireland: Report of the Trauma Steering Group* for the Department of Health, Ireland.

Positions include teaching faculty at the Royal College of Surgeons of England (RCSEng) in addition to Director of the RCSEng Definitive Surgical Trauma Skills course and a contributing author to e-Learning for Healthcare, NHS Health Education England. He is a clinical lecturer in surgery at the Royal College of Surgeons in Ireland (RCSI) and a senior clinical lecturer in surgery at University College Cork (UCC) and an honorary lecturer in surgery at Imperial College, London. He is an intercollegiate examiner in vascular surgery and the author of one other award-winning vascular textbook. He regularly lectures internationally, including visiting professorship to the University of Athens on disaster and conflict medicine.

Interests include; trauma education, trauma systems development, trauma protocol development, management of penetrating injury, complex aortic disease, complex lower limb revascularisation, pharmacological suppression of neointimal hyperplasia, vascular trauma, management of non-compressible haemorrhage, pelvic trauma, trauma thoracotomy, management of postpartum haemorrhage, biomarkers for shock and haemorrhage and management of the open abdomen, including abdominal wall reconstruction.

Contributors

John H. Armstrong, MD FACS
Trauma Network Director and
Associate Professor of Surgery
University of South Florida,
Tampa, Florida
and
Former Florida Surgeon General
and Secretary of Health
Tallahassee, Florida

**Mark W. Bowyer Col (ret), MD
FACS DMCC FRCS (Glasg)**
Ben Eiseman Professor of Surgery
The Uniformed Services
University and Walter Reed
National Military Medical Center
Bethesda, Maryland

Daniel Grabo, MD FACS
Associate Professor of Surgery
West Virginia University
Morgantown, West Virginia

**Mansoor Khan, MBBS PhD
FRCS FEBS AKC FACS**
Surgeon Commander Royal Navy
Consultant Trauma and Military
Surgeon
St Mary's Hospital Major
Trauma Centre
London, United Kingdom

**Morgan McMonagle, MB BCh
BAO (Hons) MD FRCSI FACS**
Consultant General
and
Trauma and Vascular Surgeon
St Mary's Hospital Major
Trauma Centre
London, United Kingdom

and

The South/South West Hospital
Group
University Hospital Waterford
Waterford, Ireland

**Jonathan J. Morrison, PhD
FRCS**
Assistant Professor of Surgery
R Adams Cowley Shock Trauma
Center
University of Maryland Medical
System
Baltimore, Maryland

**David M. Nott, OBE DSc MD
FRCS DMCC**
Professor of Conflict Surgery
Imperial College London
and
Consultant Vascular and Trauma
Surgeon
St Mary's Hospital Major Trauma
Centre
London, United Kingdom

James V. O'Connor, MD FACS
Professor of Surgery
University of Maryland School
of Medicine
and
Chief of Thoracic and Vascular
Trauma and Critical Care
R Adams Cowley Shock Trauma
Center
University of Maryland Medical
System
Baltimore, Maryland

Patrick Reilly, MD FCCP FACS
Professor of Surgery
Division of Trauma and Surgical
Critical Care
Perelman School of Medicine
Philadelphia, Pennsylvania

Thomas M. Scalea, MD
Physician-in-Chief
R Adams Cowley Shock Trauma
Center
University of Maryland Medical
System
Baltimore, Maryland

C. William Schwab, MD FACS
Emeritus Professor of Surgery
Division of Trauma and Surgical
Critical Care
Perelman School of Medicine
Philadelphia, Pennsylvania

Philip J. Wasicek, MD
R Adams Cowley Shock Trauma
Center
University of Maryland Medical
System
Baltimore, Maryland

1 The Philosophy of Damage Control

Daniel Grabo, Patrick Reilly and C. William Schwab

In a mature trauma system, characterised by rapid pre-hospital response times and aggressive resuscitation therapy, patients previously deemed unsalvageable will present alive to the operating theatre. However, when the historical 'norm' of complete and definitive surgery is applied to this subset, who are already hypothermic, coagulopathic and acidotic at presentation (i.e. metabolically exhausted), the shock quickly approaches an irreversible state as prolonged exposure of open surfaces and cavities disrupt further thermoregulation with additional blood loss. This additional bleeding from all raw surfaces, combined with hypoperfusion leads to organ failure. Thus, the 'lethal triad of trauma' is aggravated by the surgeon's futile attempt to fix all injuries in a single setting.

Ushering in a new approach, which introduces an alternative philosophy to such a patient, where the aims are re-focused on keeping the severely injured patient alive no matter the cost, has become the new overriding principle. This somewhat unconventional approach abandons the single, definitive surgical plan. Instead, the major compelling issues of *haemorrhage control* and *contamination containment* are addressed through abbreviated surgical techniques.

Historical background

This alternative strategy of avoiding futile definitive repair has a definite historical precedence. Although not specifically defined or codified as *damage control surgery* for trauma until the 1990s, military surgeons documented cases of packing bleeding sites to control haemorrhage in earlier times. Pringle in 1908 packed liver wounds to achieve haemostasis in addition to clamping the porta hepatis for hepatic inflow control that now bears his name. More recently, another surgical great, Halstead, utilised packing liver lacerations with non-absorbable materials for the same purpose. These abbreviated surgical techniques of liver packing for haemostasis after trauma, however, remained aloof and out of 'mainstream' practice for many years, until Lucas and Ledgerwood again described its utility in a small number of patients. A few years later, Harlen Stone in 1983 described abbreviated laparotomy and packing after major abdominal trauma. In this series, 76% of patients who underwent abbreviated laparotomy and packing for trauma survived as compared with only 1 out of 14 undergoing definitive repair at the index operation.

Redefining the paradigm

In 1993, Rotondo and Schwab described the damage control approach after trauma to an abbreviated procedure (laparotomy) to control bleeding and contamination, followed by aggressive resuscitation in the intensive care unit (ICU) with a planned return to the operating theatre for definitive repair of injuries (i.e. avoiding complete and definitive surgery at the index procedure). This generated a paradigm shift in the approach to the severely injured patient that is now considered the modern standard of practice. Other alternative terms in the vernacular include 'staged', 'abbreviated' and 'bail-out' surgery.

Despite the terms 'abbreviated' and 'bail-out', damage control surgery (DCS) is not a 'can't fix, won't fix' approach, but is in fact a well-thought-out and planned management attack, influenced by the measured (both quantitative and qualitative) injury burden and patient physiology and even considers the demands placed on the team, facility and system at the time (i.e. the *predicted clinical course*). The goal of DCS is to create a stable anatomical environment in which haemorrhage and contamination are rapidly controlled, thereby halting progression of the patient's physiology to an unsalvageable metabolic and physiologic state. Once an anatomically stable environment has been achieved with rapid control of bleeding, the trauma team can then turn attention to correcting the hypothermia, acidosis and coagulopathy with continued resuscitation in a more controlled and conducive environment (i.e. ICU, as stage II of DCS).

Lethal triad of trauma

The lethal triad of trauma is a vicious cycle cascade of self-perpetuating physiologic changes that result after massive haemorrhage and severe tissue trauma. Additional 'hits' (often iatrogenic) to the stressed physiologic milieu include fluid administration, operative exposure, further tissue injury from prolonged surgery and packed red blood cell (PRBC) administration. The ability to adequately perfuse the tissues and generate clot formation is lost with poor oxygen delivery and intravascular volume support. This loss of clotting factors from haemorrhage becomes further aggravated. Hypothermia results from blood loss (heat-carrying tissue) in addition to prolonged exposure of the patient and open body cavities by heroic efforts in the operating suite to control injuries. This in turn can lead to fatal arrhythmias, platelet dysfunction and further traumatic coagulopathy. Consumptive or depletion coagulopathy develops and worsens non-surgical bleeding, which although may be aggravated by fluid administration, it is also directly associated with injury severity with a linear mortality relationship. Ultimately, continued hypovolaemic shock and poor tissue perfusion generates an overwhelming anaerobic demand and resulting acidosis. The three elements to the lethal triad of trauma of *hypothermia*, *coagulopathy* and *acidosis* are all interdependent, but also each one is individually prognostic of a poor outcome, as they reflect the magnitude of injury and shock and ultimately recoverability.

Damage control defined

Damage control is as much a philosophy as a technique that, when best applied, *guides the resuscitation* for the most severely injured patients. From the time care is first rendered in the pre-hospital setting with rapid transportation to deliver the patient to the trauma centre, damage control concepts guide the trauma team to deliver best care. Damage control starts in the pre-hospital field and emergency department (ED) where simple measures to halt bleeding (compressible haemorrhage) and resuscitation begin. This pre-operative phase should be as brief as possible and is often referred to as stage 0 DCS. The next phase (especially for non-compressible cavity bleeding: thorax, abdomen–pelvis) continues as an abbreviated initial operation to grossly and expeditiously control haemorrhage and contamination (stage I DCS), which is then followed by a longitudinal and continuous resuscitation phase in the ICU (stage II DCS) where physiologic normality is restored (i.e. reversing the triad). Finally, there is a return to the operating room for definitive surgery (Stage III DCS), avoided during stage I, including formal closure of the abdomen, which typically encompasses the final phase (**Figure 1.1**).

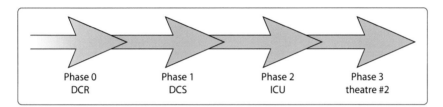

| Phase 0 | Phase 1 | Phase 2 | Phase 3 |
| DCR | DCS | ICU | theatre #2 |

Figure 1.1 Damage control pathway. The minority of patients who present to the ED trauma resuscitation area are candidates for damage control and follow the pathway of damage control resuscitation, abbreviated initial surgery, continued resuscitation in the ICU, and finally definitive surgical care.

DCS is not appropriate for every trauma patient, as the vast majority of patients seen by the trauma team who require operative intervention will follow the conventional and usual pathway (i.e. they do not fit the criteria reflective of an exhausted milieu or risk of developing one). After a traumatic event, pre-hospital providers engage appropriate interventions with rapid transportation to a trauma centre. Upon arrival, the trauma team quickly initiates resuscitative efforts in parallel with making a diagnosis utilising appropriate adjuncts. **Resuscitation includes haemorrhage control as appropriate**. This is typically followed by proceeding to definitive repair in the operating theatre, followed by recovery in the appropriate clinical setting. For a small minority (5%–15%) of severely injured patients, or those who find themselves in unique situations (mass casualty), this approach is not best practice and is even harmful. These patients require a damage control pathway, starting pre-hospital, aimed at controlled resuscitation and abbreviated surgical intervention in the early phases.

The goal of damage control resuscitation (DCR) and DCS is to prevent or limit the lethal triad to preserve the living patient. Specifically, DCR targets the global ischaemic state and coagulopathy, and addresses the metabolic derangements caused by bleeding and subsequent tissue ischaemia. In addition to appropriate and controlled resuscitation, DCS aims to control surgical bleeding rapidly and minimise contamination while postponing definitive repair pending restoration of physiology. The patient who most likely will benefit from damage control is also the one who will likely need a massive blood transfusion. Patients with three out of four of the factors presented in **Figure 1.2** have 70% predicted risk of requiring a massive transfusion and an 85% risk if all four are present.

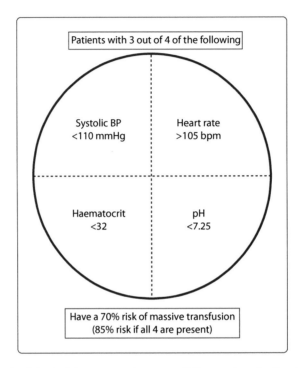

Figure 1.2 Certain physiological derangements are predictive markers for the development of both the 'trauma triad of death' and/or the need for massive transfusion. These include: BP <110mmHg, heart rate >105, haematocrit <32 and pH <7.25. If three of these factors are deranged simultaneously, there is a 70% risk of such and an 85% risk if four are deranged respectively. Additional risk factors include; injury pattern (penetrating chest or abdomen), admission INR (>1.4), O_2 saturations <75% and a base deficit >6mEq/L.

The decision to apply DCR and DCS should be made early and aggressively, even pre-emptively before surgery has begun, by recognising the deranging physiologic parameters, significant injury burden, and/or the need for massive blood transfusion. *The more hesitant the surgeon and the later damage control is applied, the less successful the outcome.* Avoid delay and deliberation!

Phases of damage control

Phase 0 DCS: The pre-surgery phase

Damage control begins by recognising and identifying the massively injured patient in the field and/or trauma bay. This may be considered a 'pre-surgical' phase. At this point the members of the trauma team (including pre-hospital providers, emergency physicians and trauma surgeons) must recognise those patients with a large injury burden and significant physiologic derangement in addition to massive blood transfusion requirements and instigate DCR.

A key early concept during phase 0 is to control or limit compressible haemorrhage (e.g. apply tourniquets [TKs]) and pelvic binders as appropriate, and manage open bleeding wounds by packing with haemostatic agents and compression dressings. Chest tube placement will help reduce pleural space bleeding and rapid 'whip' suturing to lacerations may also be appropriate.

Lessons learned on the battlefields of Iraq and Afghanistan, have translated to the civilian pre-hospital community, including the implementation of protocols and training for the use of limb tourniquets in extremity haemorrhage. Additionally, pre-hospital providers are becoming more adept and well trained in the use of pelvic binding devices and haemostatic wound packing agents. The concept of 'permissive hypotension' has now been adopted into our pre-hospital service, as injured patients are now transported with a lower blood pressure than was historically treated, as long as they maintain evidence of adequate end-organ perfusion (e.g. central pulse, awake and talking) *in lieu* of performing time-consuming interventions in the field, such as copious administration of intravenous (IV) fluids. Rapid transportation to a trauma centre, instead of intervening in the field, is associated with a significant decrease in time to surgical control of bleeding, which is the *single best predictor of a successful outcome* and also results in less fluid and blood product transfusion (and the risks associated with these).

Once haemorrhage control has been achieved (that is manageable in the field or trauma bay), the team must then rapidly progress through the trauma evaluation *as per* ATLS™ guidelines. Minimal adjunctive testing is necessary (e.g. CXR, PXR, FAST exam), aimed at only seeking out occult haemorrhage or to guide the team to the likely compelling source of cavity bleeding. After a rapid assessment, decision-making must be timely, expeditious and definitive based on the information gathered from the assessment and patient parameters. This serves to inform the commencement of resuscitation. However, *you cannot successfully resuscitate the actively bleeding patient!* Until surgical (or angiographic) control of haemorrhage is achieved, the guiding principle of the initial phase of damage control is 'haemostatic resuscitation', and the damage control pathway is instigated.

Damage control measures at this stage include minimising crystalloid fluid infusions and instead utilising blood and blood product transfusion to resuscitate to an 'adequate' (i.e. survivable) blood pressure and perfusion. If a blood transfusion is required, the transfusion should be delivered with plasma and platelets in a tight ratio of 1:1:1 (PRBC to plasma to platelets), which has been shown to improve survival and is supported by both military and civilian studies. The activation of a *massive transfusion protocol*, where all blood components are delivered to the patient's bedside (theatre, ED, ICU) with the proper ratios described and in rapid succession has been shown to deliver blood more effectively and efficiently, with fewer complications. The inclusion of cryoprecipitate provides additional fibrinogen, which is deficient in plasma. Additional dynamic information on the patient's coagulation profile can be learned from bedside testing such as thromboelastography. Tranexamic acid, an inexpensive antifibrinolytic agent, has also been shown in large studies in both civilian and military trauma patients to improve survival when given early (1 g bolus followed by 1 g infusion over 8 hours within 3 hours of injury) to patients requiring massive blood transfusion.

Phase I DCS: The surgical phase

When the key physiological parameters of severe haemorrhage or injury are present or expected (pH <7.25, base deficit <6, core temperature <36°C, international normalised ratio [INR] >1.4, haemoglobin [Hb] <11 g/dL, heart rate [HR] >105 bpm, systolic blood pressure [SBP] <110 mmHg) and/or there has been a suspected significant blood loss and coagulopathy, the decision for DCR–DCS should be made early and/or pre-emptively. This consists of (in descending order)

1. Haemorrhage control
2. Contamination control
3. Intra-abdominal packing
4. Temporary abdominal closure

Haemorrhage control

Haemorrhage control is initially achieved *via* rapid entry into the abdomen (or other bleeding cavity) in a standard, midline incision from the xiphoid process to the pubic bone. This incision is made sharply with skin knife and heavy scissors only in the interests of time. Upon entering the abdomen, whatever tamponade was present will be lost and the patient may experience further haemodynamic collapse. It is important to notify the anaesthetic team so that they can prepare large volume blood resuscitation. We advise having more than one suction device in use in the surgical field. Large handheld retractors to retract open the abdominal side walls are employed to allow for effective haemorrhage control by tightly packing of all four quadrants in a systematic fashion starting at the site with the most obvious source of bleeding first. If the compelling source of bleeding presents itself, such as a liver laceration or mesenteric artery bleed, it should be dealt with expeditiously. If the source is not immediately identifiable, the surgical team must proceed with a stepwise and systematic approach to evaluate the abdomen, but we advocate beginning at the left upper quadrant (LUQ) (as the spleen is statistically the most likely source of intra-abdominal haemorrhage) and working clockwise. We advocate the following approach:

1. Pack all four quadrants as detailed earlier (**Figure 1.3**).
2. Examine zone 1 of the retroperitoneum. This is the zone containing the aorta and is below the transverse mesocolon, best visualised initially by eviscerating the small bowel to the patient's right-hand side. The surgeon can then decide if total inflow control to the abdomen is required.
3. In a systematic fashion remove the packs from the four quadrants examining the solid organs (spleen, liver, kidneys) as well as zone 2 of the retroperitoneum bilaterally. We advocate to start by removing the packs from the least compelling source of bleeding first to aid in declaring these areas 'injury-free'. Finally, remove packs from zone 3 in the pelvis.

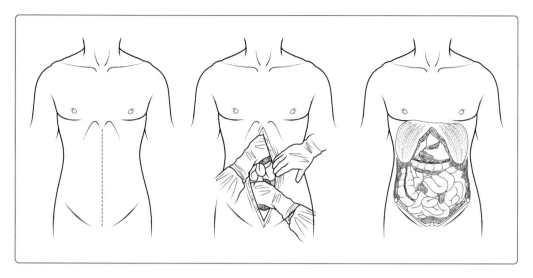

Figure 1.3 Intra-abdominal packing. Demonstration of packing control of haemorrhage. Rolled up (for added tamponade) large abdominal packs are placed systematically into the left upper quadrant and followed in a clockwise direction along the left paracolic gutter. The pelvis is also packed above the peritoneal reflection (additionally extraperitoneal pelvic packing is utilised if an expanding pelvic haematoma is also present). Packing is continued along the right paracolic gutter and finally the liver is packed into its normal anatomical shape (above, below and laterally).

4. Run the entire small bowel from the ligament of Treitz to the cecum. Then completely evaluate all aspects of the colon from caecum to rectum and inspect all colonic wall haematomas. Be sure to inspect the mesentery down to its root looking for bleeding and haematoma, and the transverse colon underneath the greater omentum.
5. Finally, inspect the stomach (anterior and posterior surfaces). Be sure to open the lesser sac to inspect the posterior gastric surface (and gastro-oesophageal junction) and evaluate the pancreas as well. Kocherise the duodenum to inspect it front and back and the head of pancreas front and back.

It is best to deal with and manage serious injury contemporaneously as it is encountered whilst at the same time prioritising each by the most compelling source of bleeding first (which can be challenging with multiple bleeding sites).

1. Solid organ injury
   a. *Liver – Therapeutic packing* is typically sufficient for the majority of liver injuries. By approximating the injured or cut edges of liver into its *normal anatomical configuration* and into the normal liver bed with packs will control the majority of hepatic bleeding. Additional techniques to control hepatic vascular inflow (i.e. *Pringle manoeuvre*) by clamping the hepatic artery and portal venous inflow in the free edge of the lesser omentum are used if not sufficiently controlled with therapeutic packing alone or if the liver requires further mobilisation for large posterior bleeding. Retro-hepatic venous injuries are preferably left undisturbed if they are

adequately controlled with packing. Otherwise, a combination of Pringle manoeuvre with or without *total hepatic vascular isolation* (additional supra- and infra-hepatic inferior vena cava [IVC] control, with or without individual isolation of the hepatic veins as they exit the liver posteriorly and directly into the retro-hepatic IVC) can significantly decrease liver bleeding while uncontrollable retro-hepatic venous injuries are addressed (liver is mobilised forwards by taking down the right and left triangular ligaments as necessary). An additional sub-costal skin incision and/or splitting the diaphragm (circular through the muscular portion) will dramatically improve exposure for these lethal injuries. Other techniques for hepatic lacerations include large, deep liver sutures (with or without an omentum pedicle plug), balloon tamponade of missile tract injuries, or the addition of commercially available haemostatic agents can be useful in difficult-to-control injuries (see Chapter 9).

    b. Spleen and kidney – In true damage control, where the patient is exsanguinating from an injury to either the spleen or kidney, there is little room for splenic or renal preservation. Thus, the DCS option is splenectomy and nephrectomy, respectively.

    c. Pancreas – Devastating injury to the tail of the pancreas (i.e. left of the superior mesenteric vessels) is best addressed with distal pancreatectomy using a stapling device followed by wide drainage of the injured field. A concomitant splenectomy is typically also necessary. Pancreatic head injuries (i.e. to the right of the superior mesenteric vessels) are best controlled with packing and drain placement initially unless deemed to be devastating and involving the duodenum for which a trauma Whipple's resection is best. This is associated with a very high mortality and best done as a staged procedure (if gross haemorrhage is controlled at the index operation). Of course, reconstruction post-resection is deferred until take back (DCS stage III).

2. Major vascular injury

    a. Simple, direct repair is often the best and fastest method of achieving both haemorrhage control of a major vascular injury whilst restoring forward perfusion (**Figure 1.4**). Of course, attention to appropriate wound edge debridement and approximation (especially tunica intima) is important (to avoid 'flap' creation and thrombosis).

    b. Ligation may be necessary in the exsanguinating patient. For certain large vessels (e.g. infra-renal inferior vena cava (IVC), inferior mesenteric artery (IMA), coeliac artery (CA), there may be an acceptable morbidity. However, other vessel ligations are associated with a near 100% mortality regardless (e.g. aorta, superior mesenteric artery [SMA]).

    c. Temporary vascular shunts are the most useful vascular damage control adjunct (by controlling bleeding and preserving perfusion), and their benefit has been demonstrated in both extremity vascular trauma and in major vascular injuries to the carotid and the named mesenteric vessels.

3. Raw surface bleeding

    a. Therapeutic packing is often all that is required to control raw surface haemorrhage (from either the initial injury or the surgical dissection) especially in the coagulopathic patient.

    b. Additional haemorrhage control may be achieved with the use of commercially available haemostatic agents.

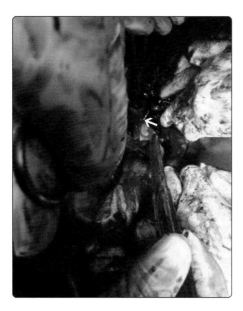

Figure 1.4 Major vascular injury. Sponge stick control of an isolated infra-renal IVC injury (arrow) that was repaired primarily with running 4-0 non-absorbable suture.

4. Pelvic bleeding
   a. First and foremost, restore *pelvic volume* to normal with binders and pelvic compression devices (e.g. external fixation to significantly decrease blood loss volume). These should be reserved for certain fracture patterns, such as the open book pelvis, that warrant pelvic compression, to restore the normal anatomical volume of the pelvis and provide tamponade.
   b. Pelvis-only preperitoneal packing (when the injury and bleeding is confined to the pelvis only) is best done through a midline incision taking great care to avoid entering the peritoneal cavity. As the preperitoneal space is developed, the large pelvic haematoma is evacuated and the space packed with laparotomy pads. If a laparotomy is already in progress (typically for other bleeding injuries), then the preperitoneal packing may be performed through the same incision by stripping the peritoneal reflection off the pelvic sidewall (often the haematoma has done this for you!) and packing deep into the pelvic cavity with large laparotomy pads.
   c. Temporary internal iliac artery occlusion (vascular loops and clamps) is best achieved during formal laparotomy and serves to achieve control of extravasation from the internal iliac (hypogastric) arteries and to decrease inflow into the pelvis. The vessel loops can then be let down after haemostasis is achieved days later.
   d. Angioembolisation is an extremely useful adjunct in pelvic trauma where a contrast extravasation blush is seen on angiogram (e.g. computed tomography angiography [CTA]), as it can arrest haemorrhage deep inside the 'hard to reach' parts of the pelvis. It may be used after laparotomy and packing.
5. Contamination control
   a. Contamination control is best achieved with simple techniques to stop and contain leaks from any hollow viscus injury (gastric, small bowel, colonic). Techniques

including simple sutures, umbilical tapes, gastrointestinal (GI) staplers and bowel clamps can effectively control spillage from the GI tract. It is best to leave the bowel ends in discontinuity during contamination control (if a rapid resection has been performed) rather than to attempt a formal resection and anastomosis (which is likely to dehisce and leak in the shocked patient). The bowel will likely develop an ileus and the risk of perforation in the discontinuous segment within a few days is minimal. Additionally, simple suture repair of a bladder injury will control urine leaks. Defer definitive GI and genitourinary (GU) tract repair, which may involve resection and anastomosis until time of take-back. Of note, it is important to *place drains in dependent areas where bile, pancreatic or urinary contents may collect* as these are not well controlled by abdominal vacuum suction devices on closure and can lead to significant inflammation that may hinder the definitive operation at take-back.

Closure

It is important to re-address *intra-abdominal packing* once more to ensure that all raw surfaces are effectively packed. Typically, if packing is effective, the top abdominal packs should be white (i.e. not soaked in blood). Additionally, take the time to inspect all the concerning injuries that were controlled with packing or any other means of haemorrhage control to be certain that nothing major was missed or ineffectively controlled. An early take-back to the operating suite because of failure to control the haemorrhage at the index operation is associated with a higher mortality and morbidity.

By the time this initial (index) operation is complete the patient will likely have experienced (in addition to massive intra-abdominal injury), a massive blood transfusion (with its side effects and risks) and potentially reperfusion injury (from shock and/or clamping). Therefore, massive oedema within the abdomen and its domain are expected, despite restrictive use of crystalloids during resuscitation. With potential loss of domain, forcing an abdomen closed is a set up for disaster including abdominal compartment syndrome and massive dehiscence (burst abdomen). Avoid fascial sutures at this point!

Temporary closure

Temporary closure is best achieved using a commercially available or hand-fashioned vacuum suction device (**Figure 1.5**). The principles are the same. After achieving haemostasis and controlling contamination, packs are strategically placed in the abdomen especially on raw surfaces to compress solid organs. Additional drains are placed in dependent portions of the abdomen especially after hepato-biliary or genito-urinary injury, including both paracolic gutters and the pelvis. A plastic sheet, which is ideally fenestrated, is then placed over the visceral contents. White towels or a commercial sponge is then placed on top of the fenestrated plastic sheet. If a homemade device is being fashioned, then suction drains are placed over the towels and covered by an additional plastic sheet (e.g. Ioban™). Commercially available devices do not typically require additional suction drains. These temporary closure techniques allow additional abdominal tamponade, manage drainage output and herniation of visceral contents in addition to being easier to nurse the patient in the critical care setting.

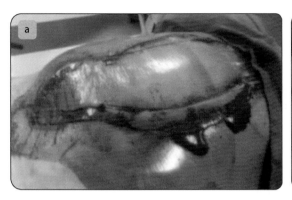
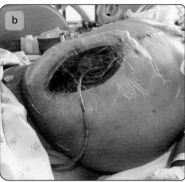

Figure 1.5 Temporary abdominal closure. Examples of different options for temporary abdominal closure. (a) The abdomen has been strategically packed and drained and a non-porous adhesive device (e.g. Ioban™) is placed on top of the open abdomen to generate a temporary closure (which is also compliant). (b) The commercially available Abthera™ device has been placed in the abdomen (sponge element) with its adherent temporary closure stretched over it and a suction device placed *in situ* to generate a negative pressure vacuum closure of the abdomen.

After closure

There is increasing use of interventional radiology (IR) and angioembolisation (AE) for haemorrhage control in trauma surgery, including a growing use in DCS. Consideration should be given for the use of IR and AE in the case of a well-packed or temporary controlled liver and pelvic bleeds (as these are challenging to access surgically) during or immediately after the initial DCS. If the patient 'normalises' or becomes near normal with ongoing resuscitation they can go the IR suite or be taken to the hybrid operating room for AE (liver, pelvis) immediately after DCS or sometime later.

Phase I of DCS should take *no more than 90 minutes* from time of arrival in the operating theatre until the time the patient is packaged up and ready to leave for the ICU. Ideally, the decision for DCS will have been made early after recognising the key physiologic parameters and presenting characteristics that necessitate it in the first place. Upon arrival in theatre, the team will have already been instructed on and planned for an abbreviated operation that focuses on haemorrhage and contamination control with optimal communication between all team members for adequate resuscitation with massive blood transfusion in proper prescribed ratios and appropriate adjuncts. Resist the urge and temptation to 'fix everything' in these patients, as definitive repair is likely doomed to failure with certain death of the patient!

Phase II DCS: The resuscitation phase

At the completion of phase I, the patient is transferred directly to the ICU for the following:

1. Rewarm utilising core rewarming techniques.
2. Correct coagulopathy with blood products. Where available viscoelastic testing can be used to guide choice of blood products.
3. Correct acidosis by attention to maximising haemodynamics and optimising ventilation and oxygenation (and not by artificially enhancing the pH with alkalanising agents).

As the patient stabilises (the physiologic and metabolic parameters will trend towards normal over several hours), additional studies (x-rays, CT scans, contrast enhanced studies) can be performed to identify additional injuries (e.g. spinal, traumatic brain injury [TBI]) or to better characterise those already known. This is also an ideal time to recruit the expertise of consultants for additional management and definitive repairs, especially if a subspecialist is required (e.g. vascular, urology, pelvic [acetabular] surgeon).

It is imperative to monitor the patient for the development of *abdominal compartment syndrome* (ACS). Despite having an 'open' abdomen, the patient is still at risk (albeit less so) from massive fluid shifts, ongoing resuscitation, missed injury or reperfusion injury. Both homemade or commercial devices are available to monitor bladder pressures which when above 15-20 mmHg are concerning for ACS, but certainly raised intra-abdominal hypertension (IAH). Other parameters including hypotension, acute renal insufficiency (especially oliguria) and raised airway pressures (peak inspiratory pressure and mean airway pressure) are indicative of ACS and should be addressed. Management should include an exhaustive search for the cause, which can range from medical management (including sedation and paralysis, diuresis) to surgical (re-exploration to search for a missed injury, ongoing bleeding or just abdominal decompression to relieve the IAH). ACS is not something to be taken lightly as its development in the damage control abdomen is associated with a significantly higher mortality.

Phase III DCS: The relook with or without formal abdominal closure phase

When the patient's physiological numbers normalise and blood and product requirements cease with a return to normothermia, they are then ready to go back for definitive repair. This usually takes 12–72 hours. If during the initial hours in the ICU (after phase 1) the patient remains hypothermic and requires ongoing blood transfusion or has a rising lactate (worsening acid-base balance), they may need an earlier-than-planned return to surgery, not for definitive repair but for re-exploration for ongoing bleeding or a missed injury (i.e. a return to DCS Stage I). Occasionally, IR is used instead if the source of the problem is deemed to be bleeding amenable to AR (with challenging surgical access).

After 12–72 hours the appropriately resuscitated patient will have met the criteria to return to theatre for definitive surgery. Returning to theatre too early (<12 hours) to remove packs can result in significant re-bleeding. Waiting too long (>72 hours) can result in sepsis rates that are too high. When removing packs, it is best to do this slowly under warm water (to avoid a dry, adherent swab from tearing clot from raw surfaces). Occasionally pre-emptive vascular control is also necessary. Additional haemostatic devices and agents such as argon beam and fibrin glue can be used after packs are removed to control minor 'ooze'. After complete exploration and inspection for additional injuries and to evaluate known injuries and repairs, definitive repairs are undertaken. For vascular injuries, both arterial and venous injuries are repaired after removal of shunts. Vein grafts and synthetic conduits can be used effectively.

After further inspection, both solid organ and bowel injuries are repaired. At this point, minimal therapy to the liver is advised as long as haemostasis remains. Ideally, stomas are avoided as much of the historical enthusiasm for stoma placement has by now been abated, as the patient is no longer receiving ongoing blood resuscitation or vasopressors, making an anastomosis more likely to heal. Thus, primary repair or anastomosis is preferred. If a stoma is necessary, it is ideal to place it lateral to the rectus (and high up), as this muscle might be necessary in abdominal wall reconstruction. Avoid feeding tubes through the abdominal wall for the same reason. Opt instead for naso-gastric or jejunal feeding tubes in the short term.

After copious irrigation and appropriate drain placement, perform primary fascial closure. Again, *do not force the fascia closed.* Primary fascial closure can be readily achieved in 80% of DCS by day 5. Leave the skin open temporarily, and plan to close this in a few days to avoid wound infection. If a tension-free fascial closure is not possible (typically if the abdomen has remained open >5 days), opt instead for planned ventral hernia with either a staged closure or more definitive anterior abdominal wall reconstruction (beyond the scope of this book).

Outcomes after DCS

Damage control surgery works! It is particularly efficacious in that sub-group of exsanguinating patients with major vascular and multiple visceral injuries. The application of DCS can also be extended to situations where the surgeon, patient, or environment demands a delay or postponement of definitive surgery, such as in mass casualty scenarios or elective surgery with intra-operative complications and a deteriorating patient.

Rotondo et al. in 1993 described an increase survival rate for those massively injured patients who underwent damage control laparotomy compared with those who had definitive management (77% versus 11%). Although this was a small subset, the results were staggering, and the concept and application of damage control laparotomy became the standard approach for the massively injured patient at the hospital of the University of Pennsylvania, before gaining popularity throughout level 1 trauma centres in the United States and beyond. With the advent of permissive hypotension, massive transfusion protocols and tight blood transfusion ratios, damage control resuscitation principles have gained traction and is now the standard of care in all modern trauma centres. When damage control resuscitation and surgery are performed in concert, survival improves dramatically.

The damage control laparotomy as a standard of care has seen increasing popularity as reported by Johnson in 2001 and Nicholas in 2003 with associated falling mortalities. This dramatic improvement in survival comes at an acceptable morbidity however. *Ventral hernias* require multiple surgeries and abdominal wall re-construction. *Fistulas* and intra-abdominal *infections* increase with the number of abdominal packs left in, the length of time the abdomen remains open and the use of negative pressure therapy. These and other complications such as *bile leaks* are readily managed through the use of non-operative techniques such as ERCP (endoscopic retrograde cholangiopancreatography) and radiographic drain placement. Sutton et al. in 2006 looked at long-term follow-up of patients who had undergone damage control laparotomy. Nearly all of the survivors had a planned ventral hernia and at 2 years follow-up 31 of 41 had been readmitted at least once during that time most commonly for infection, ventral hernia repair or fistula management. Of note, there were no mortalities associated with these readmissions. More recently, there is increasing evidence that with improved resuscitation techniques and blood product transfusion ratios, damage control surgery may become less necessary. In 2010, Guillermo et al. reported that despite performing more initial trauma laparotomies, they performed less damage control and less laparotomies overall due to fewer take-backs. This might, however, reflect an ever-improving trauma system, where severely injured and exsanguinating patients are identified early and managed immediately and aggressively with open surgery, making damage control unnecessary, as physiology has not had time to deteriorate when haemorrhage control is achieved early and aggressively. This is still within the philosophy of damage control surgery and resuscitation, even if stage I does not require packing with an open abdomen. The importance and strength of early and aggressive haemorrhage control in a well-run trauma system cannot be fully appreciated without first understanding the damage control philosophy.

Pitfalls

The biggest pitfall is a failure to recognise the patient in need of DCS or early enough in the process. Keen attention must be given to the presenting factors in the resuscitation area when the patient is first encountered. By recognising the massively injured patient who remains hypotensive and tachycardic, hypothermic and coagulopathic, despite ongoing resuscitation with blood (and blood products), one can quickly move down the *damage control pathway* without delay. It is in fact 'decision paralysis' (delay and deliberation) and poor communication that often results from failure to recognise the patient in need of damage control. Senior members of the team must pay attention to time so as not to delay moving through the process. Temperature and other key physiologic and laboratory parameters will guide the resuscitation and communicate these findings and decisions/ instructions clearly and early. Delaying patient movement between phases of DCS can easily happen due to the attempt to obtain additional information *via* radiographic studies. These can be time consuming and are often unnecessary.

DCS beyond the abdomen

The utility of DCS has also been demonstrated outside of the abdomen. Temporary vascular shunts are useful in extremity vascular injury and have been shown to improve limb viability in both military and civilian patients, (**Figure 1.6**). Damage control thoracic surgery has also been shown to be useful especially in terms of minimal lung resection,

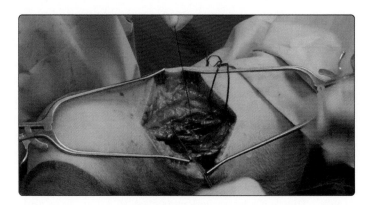

Figure 1.6 Temporary vascular shunts. Extremity vascular injury can be effectively managed in the short term with temporary shunts. Note both the vein and artery have been shunted.

as the preferred approach for lung injuries is tractotomy followed by wedge resection and non-anatomical resection as opposed to formal lobectomy.

Additional evidence exists for the use of abbreviated surgical techniques in place of definitive traditional care for orthopaedic neurosurgery including spine trauma, and non-trauma emergency abdominal surgery and other causes of major haemorrhage, including massive post-partum bleeding. Patients at the extremes of age are also candidates, as paediatrics and the elderly have been shown to be the beneficiaries of damage control surgical techniques as well.

Extended use for DCS

While there is increasing attention to DCR with potentially less frequent indications for DCS, it remains that any massively injured patient in severe shock with acidosis, hypothermia and coagulopathy will benefit from an abbreviated operation whose sole purpose is to quickly arrest haemorrhage and control contamination. Surgeon judgment also must be considered. Does the team have the ability to perform the definitive repair? Are the resources and the skill set present? Would the patient benefit more from a temporary solution until more expertise can be mobilised? Is this a scenario with multiple casualties or where the full extent of the situation is not yet known? We have learned from our colleagues in Israel that during the first 3 hours of a mass casualty event, the majority of patients requiring operative intervention will present themselves. Thus, the greatest strain to the system in terms of space, personnel and resources will usually be seen in just a few hours after the incident. These key decisions might present to the military or the civilian trauma surgeon after a mass casualty situation. It is at this time that minimal acceptable care or damage control is most appropriate until more resources are available to provide the required definitive care or until the patient can be safely transferred to a centre that can provide the necessary next stage.

Summary

Damage control is a conscious, planned therapeutic approach to resuscitation and surgery that can be applied to all surgical fields with rapid control of haemorrhage and contamination in an abbreviated fashion utilising prescribed surgical techniques. Key early components to its successful implementation include early recognition of the patient in whom DCS is mandated which is rapidly communicated and these decisions put in to the *damage control action plan*. The initial phase of the damage control operation is abbreviated with attention to haemorrhage and contamination control. After restoration of normal physiologic parameters in the ICU, definitive surgery is considered with acceptable morbidities from the initial operation. Success in damage control relies as much on effective resuscitation as on a slick haemorrhage control operation. In addition, decision-making for mass casualty situations lends itself to the use of damage control concepts or in the resource-poor environment in preparation for transfer to a more definitive care hospital.

Additional reading

Bickell W, Wall M, Pepe P et al. Immediate versus delayed fluid resuscitation for hypotensive patients with penetrating torso injuries. *NEJM* 1994;331:1105–1109.

Borgman M, Spinella P, Perkins J et al. The ratio of blood products transfused affects mortality in patients receiving massive transfusions at a combat support hospital. *J Trauma* 2007;63:805–813.

Brohi K, Singh, J, Heron, M, Coats J. Acute traumatic coagulopathy. *J Trauma* 2003;54:1127–1130.

Burlew C, Moore E, Cucxhieri J et al. Sew it up! A Western Trauma Association multi-institutional study of enteric injury management in the postinjury open abdomen. *J Trauma* 2011;70:270–273.

Cotton B, Au B, Nunez T et al. Predefined massive transfusion protocols are associated with a reduction in organ failure and postinjury complications. *J Trauma* 2009;66:41–48.

Cotton B, Gunter O, Isbell J et al. Damage control hematology: The impact of a trauma exsanguination protocol on survival of blood product utilization. *J Trauma* 2008;64:1177–1182.

CRASH-2 Collaborators. Effects of tranexamic acid on death, vascular occlusive events, and blood transfusion in trauma patients with significant hemorrhage (CRASH-2): A randomized, placebo-controlled trial. *Lancet* 2010;376:23–32.

D'Amours S, Rastogi P, Ball C. Utility of simultaneous interventional radiology and operative surgery in a dedicated suite for seriously injured patients. *Curr Opin Crit Care* 2013;19:587–593.

Dubose J, Inaba K, Barmparas G et al. Bilateral internal iliac artery ligation as a damage control approach in massive retroperitoneal bleeding after pelvic trauma. *J Trauma* 2010;69:1507–1514.

Duchesne J, Kimonis K, Marr A et al. Damage control resuscitation in combination with damage control laparotomy: A survival advantage. *J Trauma* 2010;69:46–52.

Einav S, Aharonson-Daniel L, Weissman C et al. In-hospital resource utilization during multiple casualty incidents. *Ann Surg* 2006;243:533–540.

Gracias V, Braslow B, Johnson J et al. Abdominal compartment syndrome in the open abdomen. *Arch Surg* 2002;137:1298–1300.

Guillermo H, Friese R, O'Keeffe T et al. Damage control laparotomy: A vital tool once overused. *J Trauma* 2010;69:53–59.

Halsted W. Ligature and suture material: The employment of fine silk in preference to catgut and the advantage of transfixing tissues and controlling hemorrhage—Also an account of the introduction of gloves, gutta-percha tissue and silver foil. *JAMA* 1913;40:1119–1126.

Holcomb J, Wade C, Michalek J et al. Increased plasma and platelet to red blood cell ratios improve outcome in 466 massively transfused civilian trauma patients. *Ann Surg* 2008;248:447–458.

Inaba K, Aksoy H, Seamon M et al. Multicenter evaluation of temporary vascular intravascular shunt use in vascular trauma. *J Trauma* 2016;80:359–364.

Joint Theater Trauma System Clinical Practice Guideline. Damage control resuscitation at level IIb/III treatment facilities. www.usaisr.amedd.army.mil. 11 October 2012.

Joint Trauma System Clinical Practice Guideline. Vascular injury. www.usaisr.amedd.army.mil. 12 August 2016.

Johnson J, Gracias V, Gupta R et al. Hepatic angiography in patients undergoing damage control laparotomy. *J Trauma* 2002;52:1102–1108.

Johnson J. Gracias V, Schwab C et al. Evolution in damage control for exsanguinating penetrating abdominal injury. *J Trauma* 2001;51:261–269.

Kragh J, Walters T, Baer D et al. Survival with emergency tourniquet use to stop bleeding in major limb trauma. *Ann Surg* 2009;249:1–7.

Licthe P, Kobbe P, Dombroski D et al. Damage control orthopedics: Current evidence. *Curr Opin Crit Care* 2012;18:647–650.

Loveland J, Boffard K. Damage control in the abdomen and beyond. *Br J Surg* 2004;91:1095–1101.

Lucas CE, Ledgerwood AM. Prospective evaluation of hemostatic techniques for liver injuries. *J Trauma* 1976;16:442–451.

Miller R, Morris J, Diaz J et al. Complications after 344 damage-control open celiotomies. *J Trauma* 2005;59:1365–1371.

Morrison J, Dubose J, Rasmussen T et al. Military application of tranexamic acid in trauma emergency resuscitation (MATTERs) Study. *Arch Surg* 2012;174:113–119.

Newell M, Schlitzkus L, Waibel B, White MA, Schenarts PJ, Rotondo MF et al. 'Damage control' in the elderly: Futile endeavor or fruitful enterprise? *J Trauma* 2010;69:1049–1053.

Nicholas J, Rix E, Easley K et al. Changing patterns in the management of penetrating abdominal trauma: The more things change the more they remain the same. *J Trauma* 2003;55:1095–1108.

O'Connor J, Dubose J, Scalea T. Damage-control thoracic surgery: Management and outcomes. *J Trauma* 2014;77:660–665.

Ordonez C, Pino L, Badiel M et al. The 1-2-3 approach to abdominal packing. *World J Surg* 2009;36:2761–2766.

Pringle J. Notes on the arrest of hepatic hemorrhage due to trauma. *Ann Surg* 1908;48:541–549.

Rasmussen T, Clouse D, Jenkins D et al. The use of temporary vascular shunts as a damage control adjunct in the management of wartime vascular injury. *J Trauma* 2006;61:8–15.

Remick N, Shackelford S, Oh J et al. Surgeon preparedness for mass casualty events: Adapting essential military surgical lessons for the home front. *Am J Disaster Med* 2016;11:77–87.

Rosenfeld J. Damage control neurosurgery. *Injury* 2004;35:655–660.

Rotondo MF, Schwab CW, McGonigal MD et al. 'Damage control': An approach for improved survival in exsanguinating penetrating abdominal injury. *J Trauma* 1993;35:375–383.

Sartelli M, Abu-Zidan F, Ansaloni L et al. The role of the open abdomen procedure in managing severe abdominal sepsis: WSES position paper. *WJES* 2015;10:35.

Schroll R, Smith A, McSwain N et al. A multi-institutional analysis of prehospital tourniquet use. *J Trauma* 2015;79:10–14.

Shapiro M, Jenkins D, Schwab C et al. Damage control: Collective review. *J Trauma* 2000;49:969–978.

Smith W, Moore E, Osborn P et al. Retroperitoneal packing as a resuscitation technique for hemodynamically unstable patients with pelvic fractures: Report of two representative cases and a description of technique. *J Trauma* 2005;59:1510–1514.

Stone H, Strom P, Mullins R. Management of the major coagulopathy with onset during laparotomy. *Ann Surg* 1983;197:532–535.

Stylianos S. Abdominal packing for severe hemorrhage. *J Ped Surg* 1998;33:339–342.

Sutton E, Bochicchio G, Bochicchio K et al. Long term impact of damage control surgery: A preliminary prospective surgery. *J Trauma* 2006;61:831–834.

2 Ballistics and Blast Injury

David M. Nott, Mansoor Khan and Morgan McMonagle

Unfortunately, ballistic and blast injuries are no longer solely confined to the battlefield and are now being seen in the urban hospital environment with increasing frequency. A combination of the surge in terrorist activity worldwide in addition to the wider availability of cheap firearms (esp. 9 mm handgun) in urban hotspots demands that all staff involved in the management of trauma should have a working knowledge of ballistics.

Ballistics

Physics and ballistics are juxtaposed concepts, reflecting the *energy transfer* that occurs from one source to another (e.g. the kinetic energy transfer from the moving bullet to a person or structure as it decelerates) with destruction of the physical integrity of the target. The kinetic energy (KE) is represented by the equation:

$$KE = \frac{1}{2}MV^2$$

Mass versus velocity

As per the equation above, if the mass of the missile (e.g. bullet) is doubled, then the resultant kinetic energy is also doubled. However, doubling the velocity will quadruple the kinetic energy (i.e. velocity^2). Thus, a higher missile velocity will have an even greater magnitude of effect on the amount of energy transmitted compared with increasing the mass of the missile alone, with a higher potential for tissue destruction upon striking the target.

Energy dump

The 'energy dump' of a missile, describes the energy deposited into the tissues (target) after the missile strikes (i.e. the transfer of energy as the bullet slows). The greater the energy dump (energy transfer), then the greater the tissue destruction. For example, consider a gunshot wound (GSW) with both an entry and exit point, then assuming that the mass remains the same:

$$KE = \frac{1}{2}M\left(V^2\ \text{entry} - V^2\ \text{exit}\right)$$

In this case, because the missile exited the target, not all of the energy is 'dumped' within the tissues. However, if the missile does not exit, then all the energy is 'dumped' within the tissues (as the bullet comes to a halt) with greater destruction of tissues.

This concept of energy transfer within the tissues has replaced the more historical nomenclature of 'velocity' alone when lower velocity GSW's were associated with pistols and higher velocity wounds with rifles. By comparison, the modern Magnum 0.44 handgun carries nearly the same energy as an M16 rifle! (*Table 2.1*).

Table 2.1 Energies correlating with munitions

Ammunition type	Mass (g)	Velocity at muzzle (m/s)	Kinetic energy (J)
0.22 (5.56 mm) pistol	1.8	280 (924 ft/sec)	71
9 mm Smith and Wesson	9.4	220 (726 ft/sec)	227
0.44 Remington Magnum	15.6	440 (1400 ft/sec)	1510
SA80	10	940 (3100 ft/sec)	1736
M16	3.56	965 (3184 ft/sec)	1658
AK47	8	700 (2310 ft/sec)	1960

The magnitude of energy dumped by the bullet is dependent on the retardation (*drag*) force within the specific tissue that it penetrates. In turn, further retardation forces are dependent on; the penetration depth, the velocity^2, the area of the bullet as it strikes and the density of the tissue. Low-density structures (e.g. lung, muscle, soft tissue) offer little retardation on the moving missile (less likely to slow down and dump energy) compared with higher density tissue such as the liver and bone.

Historically, the propellant used to 'propel' a lead ball from a musket was black gunpowder (originating in China the third century AD). This consisted of a mixture of sulphur, charcoal and potassium nitrate (saltpetre), which in addition to energy, produced copious amounts of smoke and residue upon burning. 1 g of gunpowder produced 2500 J of heat and 270 mL of gas with 0.5 g of carbon residue. In turn, the carbon residue often 'clogged-up' the gun barrels, thereby incapacitating them! 'Rifling' of the gun barrel was engineered by placing hollows or grooves within the barrel of the gun in an attempt to 'capture' some of this residue and mitigate its side effects. Coincidentally it was also noted that the rifling had the unexpected beneficial effect of making the lead ball more accurate. The rifling within the barrel, gave gyroscopic (rotation) stability to the missile in flight and was henceforth added to internal ballistics to render accuracy.

In 1886 'smokeless' gunpowder was invented by the French, which included nitrocellulose and nitroglycerine. In addition, it was three times more powerful than black powder and burnt to produce higher pressures (1 g produced 1 L of gas with only 0.01 g of residue). Due to its higher explosive nature within the musket rifle, metal cartridges loaded with this smokeless powder were developed with the lead bullet placed on top. However, due to the greater energy being produced, the lead bullet was prone to deforming and melting in the barrel. This in turn led to the development of the *full metal jacket* (FMJ) bullet by 1889, by covering the lead with a thin coating of a more heat-resistant metal (typically copper).

Later, the British munitions factory at the Dumdum Arsenal in India, discovered that a bullet could be made more destructive by removing part of the metallic tip, leaving a small amount of exposed lead (producing greater deformation upon striking the target with a greater energy dump). However, the original dumdum bullet was rejected due to engineering difficulties (the base of the bullet was also devoid of the outer metal jacket, thereby often leaving the metal jacket within the barrel!). Improved variations were developed independently and routinely used until 1896 in Sudan, but the original town remained its popular namesake and the so-called dumdum bullet was born (**Figure 2.1a**). These bullets crumpled upon contact (i.e. deforming bullet), thereby dumping all the energy into the target and creating very large and destructive wounds (with no exit). Protests by Germany, led to The Hague Convention of 1899, deeming these wounds to be excessive and inhumane and in violation of the laws of war, leading to the prohibition of semi-jacketed bullets in warfare, which still stands today. The laws on international conflict allow only for FMJ bullets for warring parties. From 1899 to the 1950s the so-called .303 inch which equates to a 7.7 mm × 56 mm bullet was used by most warring parties (**Figure 2.1b**). Semi-jacketed bullets are however used in non-warfare situations, such as hunting and lower-energy semi-jacketed bullets are popular with western law enforcement, so that the missile remains inside the target with a reduced risk of exit and striking an innocent bystander.

A variety of bullets may be housed on top of the same calibre cartridge, each one differing in the amount of energy transferred (**Figure 2.2**). The full metal jacket bullet will retain shape and produce a smaller track within the tissue. The partially jacketed bullet will deform ('mushroom') upon entry, creating wider track with a greater dissipation of energy (**Figure 2.3**).

Ballistics are divided into three sub-categories:

1. *Internal ballistics* – This describes the dynamics of the gun, the propellant used and the terminal velocity of the bullet within the barrel up to the point of exit.
2. *External ballistics* – This describes the trajectory of the bullet after it leaves the barrel as it travels through the air but before it strikes its target.
3. *Terminal ballistics* – This describes the effects of the bullet on the target, which we refer to as *wound ballistics*, when the target is living tissue.

Internal ballistics

When the trigger is pulled, a firing pin initiates the combustion of the white powder within the cartridge, which burns to produce an instantaneous gas expansion, thereby propelling the bullet down the rifled chamber of the barrel (**Figure 2.4**).

External ballistics

The bullet leaves the muzzle at its *muzzle velocity* but is vulnerable to both *yaw* and *spin* (the slight instability of the missile in both its short and long axis), due to the expanding gases, during flight leading to 'precession' and 'nutation' of the missile. This typically stabilises again after about 50 m, with subsequent entry into the tissue point-first. The drag within the target tissue in turn will de-stabilise the bullet further as it yaws and tumbles within the tissue itself, with slowing and further energy dump (**Figures 2.5 to 2.6**).

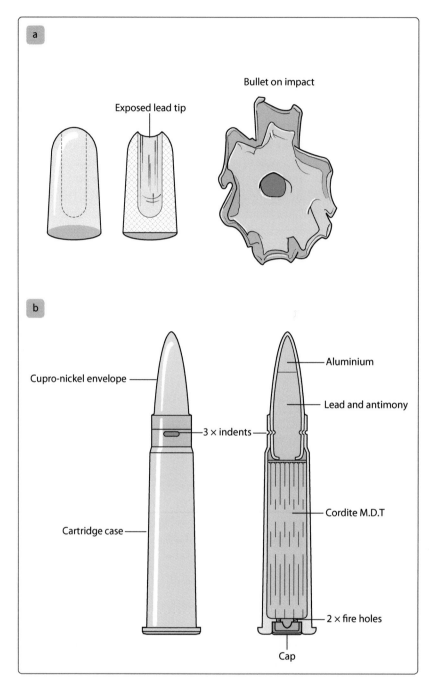

Figure 2.1 (a) Dumdum bullet. Semi-jacketed, exposing the lead tip. (b) The 0.303 inch cartridge. Most commonly used bullet in war between 1899 and 1950s.

Terminal (wound) ballistics

Wounding occurs as the bullet transfers its kinetic energy (dependent on size, mass, bullet [FMJ versus soft jacket]) casing and velocity (as described earlier). In addition, injury severity is dependent on the depth of penetration and the type of tissue struck by the missile.

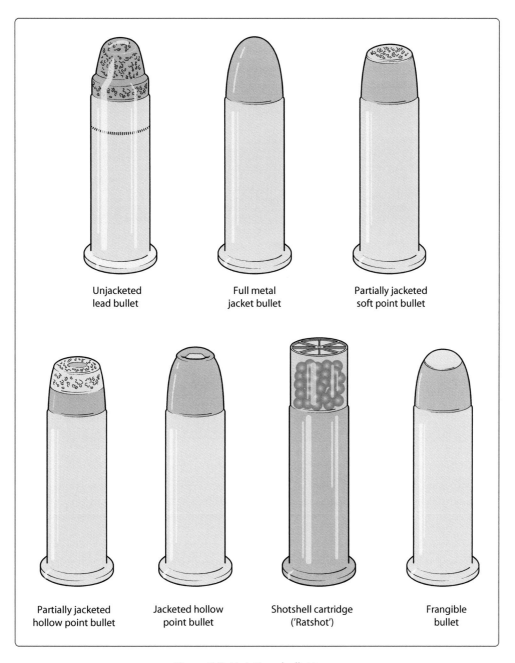

Unjacketed
lead bullet

Full metal
jacket bullet

Partially jacketed
soft point bullet

Partially jacketed
hollow point bullet

Jacketed hollow
point bullet

Shotshell cartridge
('Ratshot')

Frangible
bullet

Figure 2.2 Variations bullet types.

The pathophysiology of tissue injury occurs *via* two broad mechanisms: (1) a *permanent track* of injured or crushed tissue (reflecting the bullet trajectory within the tissue) and (2) a severe 'stretching' effect by the dissipated energy on the tissues, leading to a *temporary cavity* around (but perpendicular to) the permanent track. Typically, lower-energy bullets produce a permanent track only of direct tissue injury with no temporary cavitation effect, whereas higher-energy bullets cause more severe internal injuries due to this very high

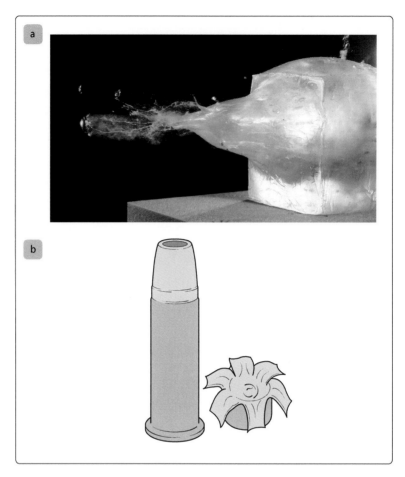

Figure 2.3 (a) A hollow tipped bullet will typically deform upon entry of the target as it 'dumps' its energy (leading to larger degrees of destruction). In this case, the bullet has also exited the target and the deformed missile is obvious. (b) An illustration of a hollow tipped bullet before and after deformation.

energy dump temporary cavity, as the energy is dissipated into the surrounding structures (remote from the permanent track).

The gel block shown in **Figure 2.3a** represents the mean human tissue density and shows a deforming bullet as it exits with greater dissipation of energy within the tissue (represented by the larger cavitation effect seen).

With lower energy missiles, death is less common unless a vital structure is hit, such as the midbrain or upper spinal cord or, more commonly, exsanguination from large blood vessel injury.

'Entry' versus 'exit' wounds

It is important that when describing a ballistic injury, never describe a wound as either 'entry' or 'exit'. This is a serious forensic matter and unless witnessed, the treating surgeon does not have any knowledge of the position of the patient (or shooter) upon being shot.

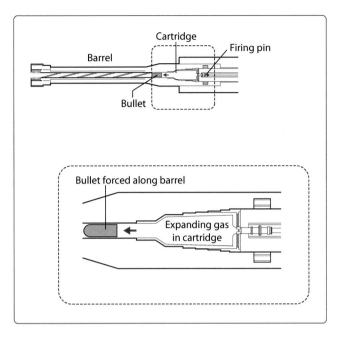

Figure 2.4 Pulling the trigger. The firing pin ignites the powder in the base of the cartridge, leading to instantaneous ignition and expansion of gases, thereby forcing the bullet (housed on top of the cartridge) out of the chamber (barrel) of the gun in rapid flight towards its target.

The size, shape and characteristics of the wounds are very dependent on patient position, angle of trajectory and type of weapon and bullet used, which is the remit of the forensic scientists (**Figure 2.7**). In addition, it is irrelevant to the immediate or operative treatment of the patient regarding which wound is an entry or an exit (or both may be entry points if shot twice or more!).

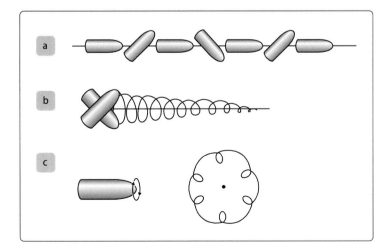

Figure 2.5 (a) Yaw: Deviation of the bullet nose away from the line of flight. (b) Precession: Rotation of the bullet around its centre of mass. (c) Nutation: Rocking of the bullet nose in the axis of rotation.

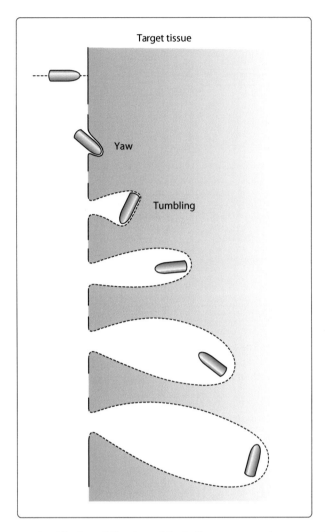

Figure 2.6 Tumble: Destabilisation of the bullet upon entering target tissue. The bullet begins to yaw and then tumbles.

Higher-energy missiles (e.g. bullet from a rifle) will produce a different pattern of injury. The high-energy missile will initially enter point first, after which it will begin to tumble (because the bullets centre of gravity is behind the centre of pressure of the bullet) inside the tissues if the trajectory track is long. With a short track, the bullet may not have time to tumble, thereby entering and exiting point first (e.g. upper limb). With longer tracks and bullet tumbling, the drag on the bullet as it presents longitudinally is the major factor in energy dissipation, thereby producing a larger, more destructive temporary cavity (**Figure 2.8**).

The temporary cavity in turn is momentarily sub-atmospheric, thereby potentially sucking additional contamination (bacteria and debris) into the wound and cavity track. Therefore, there will be a permanent track with additional high-energy temporary cavitation impinging on other surrounding structures with an additional infection risk from the combination of devitalised tissue and indrawn bacteria (**Figure 2.9**). The

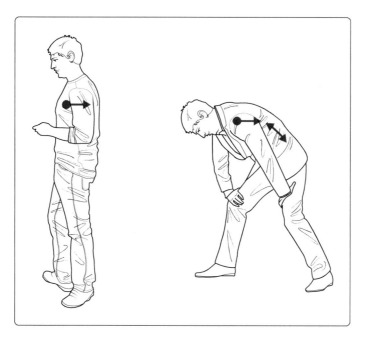

Figure 2.7 Two patients shot in the axilla. You will not know the position the patient was in when they were shot. If both patients were shot in the same area, the standing patient would probably die rapidly if the bullet traverses the heart or one of the large vessels such as the aorta. The bending patient may well survive and the bullet may end up near the pelvis as it strikes various bony structures at its final destination.

temporary cavitation effect tends to undulate for 5–10 ms^{-1} before coming to rest as the permanent track. Both positive and negative pressures alternate within the wound track, which sucks foreign material and bacteria into the track from the entrance and exit. The expanding walls of the temporary cavity are capable of doing severe damage. There is compression, stretching and shearing of the displaced tissue. Injuries to blood vessels,

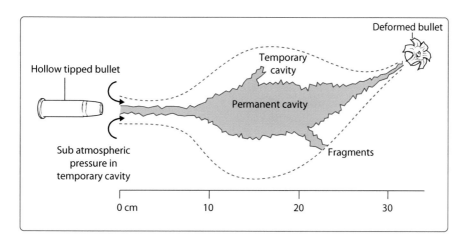

Figure 2.8 Formation of permanent tracks and temporary cavities. The sub-atmospheric temporary cavity sucks bacteria and debris into the wound.

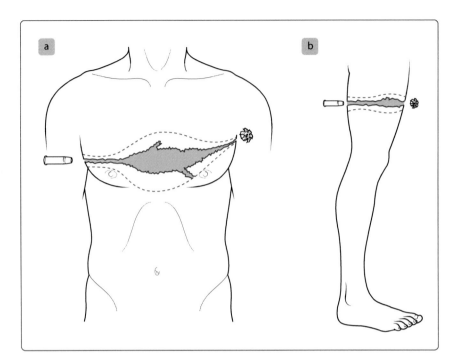

Figure 2.9 Length of wound track on formation of temporary cavity. (a) The bullet will begin to tumble inside the organ if the track is long. (b) If the track is short, then the bullet may not have time to tumble and will enter and exit point first.

nerves or organs not struck by the bullet, and a distance from the path, including bony fractures (albeit relatively rare unless directly struck by the missile). Hence, higher energy wounds tend to have higher levels of contamination and typically more aggressive debridement and wound toileting is necessary compared with lower energy wounds.

Therefore, a high-energy FMJ rifle bullet will cause tissue injury from a combination of:

- Mechanical, shredding and crushing of the tissue by the bullet as it perforates the tissue
- Shearing, compression and stretching injuries of surrounding tissue from the temporary cavitation effect
- Secondary injuries from bullet fragmentation
- Nature and density of the perforated tissue
- The length of the wound track

The size of both the temporary and permanent cavities is determined not only by the amount of kinetic energy deposited in the tissue but also by the *density* and *elastic cohesiveness* of the tissue itself. Because liver and muscle have similar densities, both tissues absorb the same amount of kinetic energy per centimetre of tissue traversed by the bullet (**Figure 2.10**). Muscle, however, has an elastic, cohesive structure; the liver is a weak, less cohesive structure. Thus, both the temporary and the permanent cavities produced in the liver are larger and more destructive than its muscular counterpart.

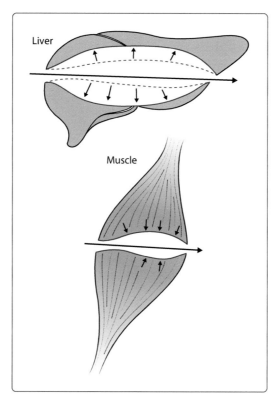

Figure 2.10 The effect of tissue structure and density on the destructiveness of the temporary cavity. Both the temporary and the permanent cavities produced in the liver are larger than those in the muscle. In muscle the tissue displaced by the temporary cavity returns to its original position. In liver the undulation of the temporary cavity disrupts the cellular supporting tissue and produces a permanent cavity approximately the size of the temporary cavity.

In muscle, the tissue displaced by the temporary cavity typically returns to its original position, with only a small rim of destruction surrounding the permanent track. In liver however, the undulation of the temporary cavity disrupts the normal tethering sites from the cellular supporting tissue, producing a large permanent cavity approximating the size of the preceding temporary cavitation. Lung however, has a very low density (specific gravity of 0.4–0.5) with a high degree of elasticity and is relatively resistant to the effects of temporary cavitation, thereby only a very small temporary cavity is typically formed with comparatively less tissue destruction.

There is, however, a critical threshold of KE dump, over which the tissue destruction becomes radically more severe. This level differs between tissues and organs. Once this KE threshold is exceeded, a temporary cavity is produced that the affected organ or tissue cannot contain (i.e. elastic limit of the organ is exceeded) and the organ 'bursts' (i.e. total destruction). This is especially destructive within the cranium as the temporary cavity forms inside the rigid skull. Therefore, brain pressure can only be relieved by bursting. Thus, a high-energy missile wound to the head tends to produce bursting injuries (**Figure 2.11**).

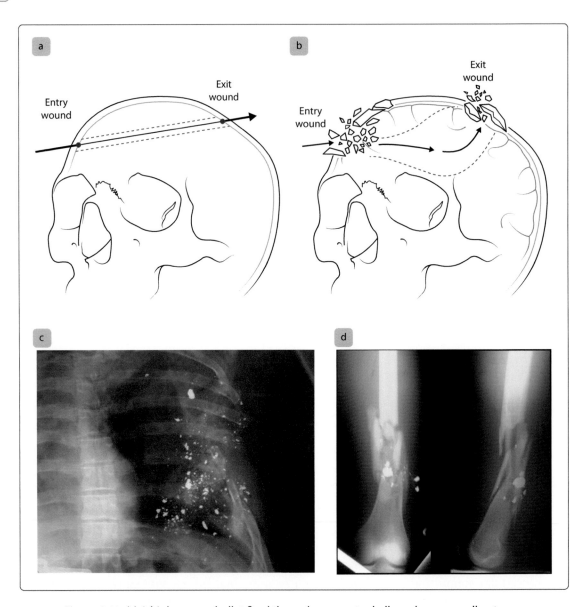

Figure 2.11 (a) A high-energy bullet fired through an empty skull produces a small entrance and exit. (b) The same missile fired through a skull containing brain causes extensive fracturing and bursting injuries. (c) Thoracic GSW with fragmentation. (d) Low-energy GSW to femur.

When a FMJ bullet strikes a hard object such as the bone, it may break up or fragment, with the lead contents acting as secondary projectiles, with the potential for increased local tissue damage (**Figure 2.11**).

Shotgun ballistics

Three types of cartridge are in common use: *birdshot* containing 1 mm pellets, *buckshot* containing 10 mm pellets, and a *slug* is a single, solid piece of lead. The lethal range for these from the average shotgun is approximately 50, 100 and 200 metres respectively. As a shotgun dissipates a large amount of its energy over a short distance (as the 'shot' dissipates rapidly), then the closer the range, the more devastating the injury (**Figure 2.12**).

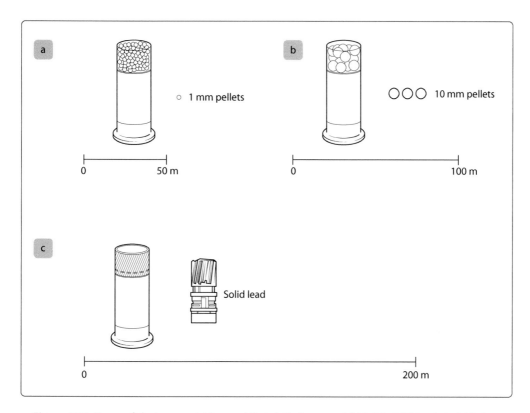

Figure 2.12 Types of shotgun cartridge and their lethal ranges: (a) birdshot (b) buckshot (c) slug.

Management of the shot victim

All exsanguinating patients must be managed with immediate surgery to the cavity or cavities where here is a compelling source of bleeding. If, however, the patient is haemodynamically well, once the primary and secondary survey have been completed and no major vascular injury is thought to exist, then the wound(s) may be directly inspected.

Low-energy bullet wounds

It can be difficult to differentiate between a high-energy and low-energy wound, but low-energy handgun bullets typically produce a path of destruction with very little lateral extension within the surrounding tissues (i.e. small temporary cavity and very little bullet fragmentation). The KE lost to the tissue is generally insufficient to cause injury remote from its track compared with higher energy missiles. Any significant injury caused by the bullet from a handgun is typically confined to a direct strike to that particular structure and its resultant permanent tract.

High-energy bullet wounds

Rifle bullets fall into two broad categories: *hunting bullets* and *military bullets*. Hunting bullets are designed to expand after impact (i.e. hollow-tipped, soft-nosed), whereas military bullets are FMJ and therefore do not. With hunting bullets, typically some fragmentation will occur and wounding is secondary to a combination of tissue crushing and shredding (as the bullet perforates the tissue), the effect of the temporary cavity with injury to tissue adjacent to the bullet path (shearing, compression and stretching) and injury from the bullet fragments. As FMJ bullets do not deform, wounding is due to the combination of tissue crush and shred (as the bullet perforates) and the effects of temporary cavitation on the surrounding structures, with additional shearing, compression and stretching. Injury due to break up of the bullet is not typically seen. The exception to this is the 5.56×45 mm (0.223) M-16 round. In addition, maximum tissue disruption with a non-fragmenting bullet will occur if the bullet strikes the target at its 'maximum surface area' (i.e. at 90° yaw to its flight path).

Remember, bullets do not respect anatomical boundaries and therefore may have traversed two or more adjacent body regions or cavities (e.g. chest to abdomen to pelvis). Examine each region carefully for wounding and especially for vascular compromise. X-ray each body region (if haemodynamics allow), as this will help identify where the bullet(s) is, if another body region has been traversed and if any bullet or bone fragmentation has occurred. X-raying each body region to account for the lodged bullet will also help the surgeon to determine the approximate trajectory of the bullet (i.e. from the surface wound to its final resting place), which in turn helps forecast the likely constellation injuries.

The projectile produces a permanent cavity containing fragments of necrotic muscle and clot. Surrounding tissue expands and stretches outwards around the path of the missile, causing a large temporary cavity of high-energy dump with zones of contusion and concussion and pockets of haemorrhage and devitalised tissue within and between muscle fibres. Temporary cavitation does not always cause a large zone of tissue damage and skeletal muscle is relatively tolerant to its effects. Thus, if a wound requires exploration, be cautious and conservative with regards to tissue excision (unless frankly necrotic) at the initial operation, as much of the tissue may still be viable and a relook(s) is always warranted.

Describing the wound

Rather misleadingly, an 'entrance' wound is described as being a circular reddish-brown margin of broken skin (i.e. abrasion ring) and an 'exit' described as being larger with stellate edges due to a combination of bullet yaw and tumble in tissue, often exiting base first or sideways (larger area) in addition to the potential for bullet deformity after entry, thereby leaving with a larger exit hole.

However, this is a misleading concept and both the entrance and exit may have differing shapes depending on many factors including; type of weapon and bullet, distance from the target, velocity of the bullet and angle of penetration. Other factors may include ricochet (before entry) or any other factor accentuating the bullet's yaw and tumble (lowering the bullet's velocity and energy pre-entry) giving a larger, ragged appearance to the entry site than expected. In addition, a fragmented bullet and deformed lead core will give a different exit wound to one which passes straight through at a higher velocity (e.g. FMJ bullet).

Therefore, *do not ascribe the wound(s) seen after a GSW as either 'entry' or 'exit'.* This is a serious medico-legal matter and should only be attempted by a forensics expert. In addition, it is irrelevant to the treatment of the patient on arrival. It is not the trauma surgeon's position to decide which wound is an entry or which is an exit (if any). *Assume all wounds are entry until proven otherwise* (with a combination of x-ray and CT scan). In addition, *all body parts must be x-rayed* as this will enable the surgeon to account for all bullets (and hence the number of times the patient has been shot) in addition to estimating the trajectory tract of the missile (by using a skin marker [e.g. paper clip] on the external wounds). *The trajectory will help to determine the expected injury pattern.*

General management of gunshot wounds

A bullet, although not sterilised by firing, is not grossly contaminated either but may carry low levels of bacteria into a wound. However, with low-velocity bullets there is less devitalised tissue destruction and the tract will seal and heal relatively quickly, rendering empirical debridement and washout unnecessary. High-energy bullets however, have a higher propensity to draw bacteria and surrounding dirt and contamination into the wound (including pieces of clothing). In addition, these wounds typically have more destruction within, with more devitalised tissue in need of debridement and washout and laying open of the bullet tract. However, *treat the wound and not the bullet.* Wounding from low-velocity bullets typically may be left, but higher-energy wounds will typically declare themselves in need of operative treatment. But, in the absence of major soft tissue injury, empirical wound exploration with laying open of the tract is typically unnecessary. Instead, the wound (if open) may be managed with dressings and allowed to drain and granulate by secondary intention, rather than direct closure and surgical exploration (which carries a higher rate of complications, including infection).

However, in a large wound with a lot of soft tissue injury and possible bony involvement, debridement may become necessary. Damaged subcutaneous fat and shredded fascia should be removed with sharp dissection and the deep fascia incised along the length of the tract or beyond to allow for adequate exploration. This also helps to relieve (or prevent) raised compartment pressures. Laying open of the tract may then be followed by irrigation with copious amounts of warm saline. Muscle is assessed for colour, consistency, contractility and capillary bleeding. Any non-viable muscle is removed and dissected back to viable (bleeding) tissue. Wounds may be left open and a surgical gauze or negative pressure dressing applied. This principal of staged treatment in grossly contaminated, necrotic and infected wounds using delayed primary closure is widely accepted with no excessive loss of skin. Wounds should be re-inspected in the operating theatre at about 48 hours and full closure planned within 4–5 days. If unable to close, a split skin graft, full thickness or even free-flap may be necessary. A few areas of skin that have sufficient vascularity such as the face, neck, scalp and genitalia may be sutured to allow primary closure but only after careful wound excision.

It is advisable to splint the injured limb for support and stabilisation using a back slab or plaster cast to protect the soft tissues even when there is no fracture. If there is a fracture, then this should be stabilised first with a back slab before assessment of the soft tissue and fracture. In the majority of unclean cases a combination of external fixation and soft tissue management will suffice.

In addition, a gunshot wound (GSW) *does not require empirical antibiotics*, unless there is a surgical reason to start (e.g. abscess, frank infection, surrounding cellulitis, etc.). If a wound does develop a complication in need of surgical treatment and antibiotics, keep in mind that the bacterial flora of the wound will change with time. In the first few days it is mainly normal skin commensals, after which both gram-positive and gram-negative wound sepsis can develop.

Bullets do not require empirical removal! It is typically safe to leave a bullet contained within the healing tract, when there are no signs of infection or necrosis (typically low-energy weapons). In fact, complication rates, including infection and secondary bleeding, are higher in studies where bullets are empirically removed. Of course, if a bullet is found during exploratory surgery for another reason (e.g. peritonitis), then it should be removed. However, *handle the bullet with rubber-shod instruments* and place in to a plastic container and hand this directly to security or law enforcement in a *chain of evidence*. Handling the bullet or grasping it with a metal instrument runs the risk of distorting the 'fingerprint' of the bullet (from the rifling of the firearm and unique to the weapon used), which may have a serious legal consequence.

There are a few exceptions to this rule however. A bullet lodged in a synovial joint should be empirically removed, as there is a theoretical risk that the continuous flow of synovial fluid through the joint may over time cause the lead to leach into the blood stream with a risk of chronic lead poisoning (*plumbism*). Besides, a bullet lodged in a synovial joint will likely give rise to symptoms and chronic fibrosis of the joint, so this in itself is a good reason to remove it before problems occur. The risk of lead poisoning probably also exists for a bullet lodged in the spinal canal (constant flow of spinal fluid) and the eye (constant flow of aqueous or vitreous fluid), although a bullet in the eye will likely lead to a destroyed eye requiring enucleation.

Gunshot wounds and fractures

Bullets striking bone can fracture it (typically comminuted fractures), but manage each case individually and on its own merit. A low-energy gunshot wound to the tibia at close range may cause a fracture with significant soft tissue damage (i.e. large energy dump), whereas a high-energy rifle bullet from a distance may cause a comminuted fracture but relatively minimal surrounding soft tissue injury.

If bone is struck by a bullet, it is highly likely that it will deform and its surrounding metal jacket will typically fragment (seen as small metallic fragments on plain x-ray and CT bony windows). In fact, if a definitive fracture is not seen after a GSW but a deformed bullet and fragmented metallic jacket is, then it is highly likely that there is also an occult fracture.

We would recommend where possible using external fixation devices (if indicated) rather than internal fixation for GSW-related bony injury to reduce further contamination and tissue injury. After a number of days, when the bullet tract is healing, this may be advanced to internal fixation at the orthopaedic surgeon's discretion.

In summary

Surgeons managing victims of gun crime need to have a working understanding of how firearms work, in particular its wounding potential so that reasonable clinical decisions can be made. It is often difficult to know whether the injury was due to a high-energy or low-energy bullet (most urban violence is low energy), but the old adage 'the surgeon should not treat the weapon' holds. Manage the soft tissue wounds and fractures similar to a non-GSW injury, but preserve as much healthy soft tissue as possible after removal of any non-viable tissue and contamination, if indicated. For massive wounds, a viable soft tissue (i.e. well-perfused soft tissue) environment must also be established, especially if a fracture is present.

Blast injuries

An *explosion* is defined as an *almost instantaneous conversion of a solid or liquid (explosive material) into a gaseous state after detonation (ignition) with the release of energy.* The generated gas expands rapidly outwards from the point (epicentre) of detonation, displacing the surrounding medium (typically air or water). This massive and rapid expansion of gas will lead to an immediate rise in pressure in the surrounding atmosphere as a blast wave, which then subsequently dissipates (degrades) over distance and time (**Figure 2.13**). There is also a lower magnitude 'sub-atmospheric' pressure wave as it degrades before the surrounding pressure returns to baseline atmospheric pressure.

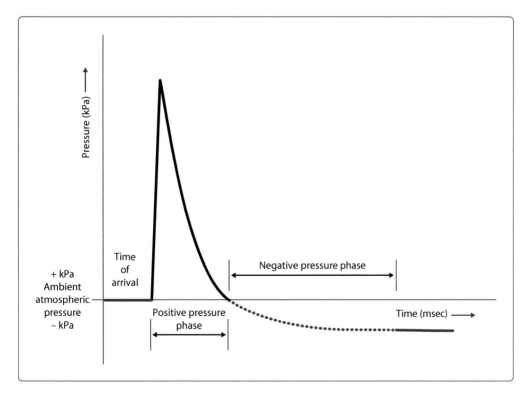

Figure 2.13 The blast wave (Friedlander waveform). There is an instantaneous over-pressurisation effect to peak pressure, before dissipation of energy occurs, which will become sub-atmospheric briefly before returning to baseline (normal atmospheric pressure).

This blast wave consists of two parts: (1) a *shock wave* of high pressure, followed closely by (2) a *blast wind* (air in motion) which can be several hundred kilometres per hour depending on the magnitude of the explosion. The blast wind will immediately propel objects or people causing injury additional to the initial shock wave (depending on proximity to the epicentre). As described earlier, the blast wave will then begin to decay immediately after its peak has been reached (*peak pressure*) followed by a *negative pressure phase* before returning to stable atmospheric pressure. The positive phase of the blast wave is characterised by *overpressure*, defined as the time between the shock arrival and the beginning of the negative phase after overpressure. *High-order* explosives such as TNT and Semtex (i.e. military grade explosives) produce a supersonic overpressure wave, whilst *low-order* explosives (e.g. gunpowder) may burn rapidly and do not produce an overpressure wave to the same extent and thus are far less destructive. The blast wave lasts for only a few milliseconds (i.e. supersonic).

Numerous factors can affect the magnitude of the blast wave. Water, which is non-compressible, will lead to a much greater potential for injury compared with air. In addition, energy delivered by the blast decreases inversely proportional to the cubed root of the distance from the epicentre of the blast. For example, the energy felt at 10 feet from the explosion delivers a blast wave 8 times more powerful than the same blast at 20 feet. Another environmental factor impacting the blast effect is whether the explosion has occurred in an enclosed or open environment. In a confined space (e.g. bus, restaurant, train) there is an amplification effect on the pressure wave as the surrounding structures confine the wave as it reverberates off walls, ceilings and so forth taking longer to decay and dissipate, maintaining above atmospheric pressure for a longer period. As a result of this confinement, the peak overpressure is raised in addition to the duration of the positive pressure phase (**Figure 2.14**).

Types of explosives

Explosives are classified as *low* order or *high* order.

Low-order explosives

Low-order explosives (e.g. gunpowder, smokeless powder, home-made explosives) burn rapidly (deflagrate) with velocities typically <1000 m/s and produce large volumes of gas that only explode if confined (e.g. a pipe bomb).

High-order explosives

High-order explosives (e.g. TNT, dynamite, Semtex) are sometimes referred to as 'military grade' and do not burn, but instead detonate when a shock wave passes through the material with velocities typically >4500 m/s leading to a substantially greater blast overpressure (**Figure 2.15**). Historical examples include the use of dynamite in the 2004 train bombing in Madrid and Semtex in the 1988 Pan Am flight 103 over Lockerbie, Scotland. Other types of explosives used include *dense inert metal explosives* (DIMEs), composed of a high-order explosive material with small particles of chemically inert material (e.g. tungsten), which are designed to produce a small but very effective explosive radius, highly lethal at close range. An *improvised explosive device* (IED) is broadly any makeshift incendiary device

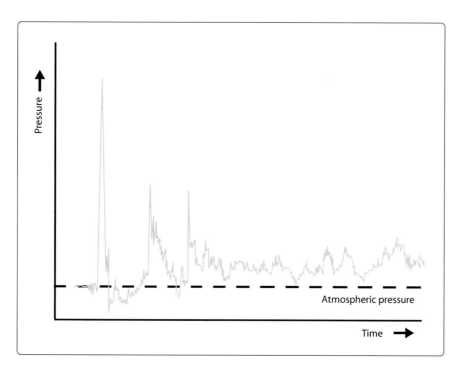

Figure 2.14 The pressure wave inside a confined space will remain over-pressurised (i.e. above atmospheric pressure) for longer (i.e. takes longer to dissipate) as it reverberates off walls, etc inside the area. The pressure waveform looks very different to the classic waveform demonstrated in **Figure 2.13**, as it consists of a multitude of mini-shock waves, taking longer to return to baseline. Confined space explosions are typically more destructive than open space ones.

constructed to explode using triggers such as mobile telephones, motion and pressure detectors.

The effect of blast injuries

Injuries caused by blast are classified into five categories: primary, secondary, tertiary, quaternary and quinary effects. However, in reality, the majority of injuries reflect a significant overlap of all categories, including in any one patient (**Figure 2.16**).

Primary blast injury

Primary blast injuries are caused by barotrauma, from either the overpressurisation or underpressurisation effect, or a combination of both. The three explosive forces leading to primary injury are *spallation*, *implosion* and *inertia*. These forces usually have a direct effect on the air–tissue interface.

Spallation
Spallation occurs when the pressure wave passes from a medium of higher density to one of lower density. For example, an explosion detonated underwater, will cause the dense water to spall into the less dense air, with fragmentation represented by the upward splash. This

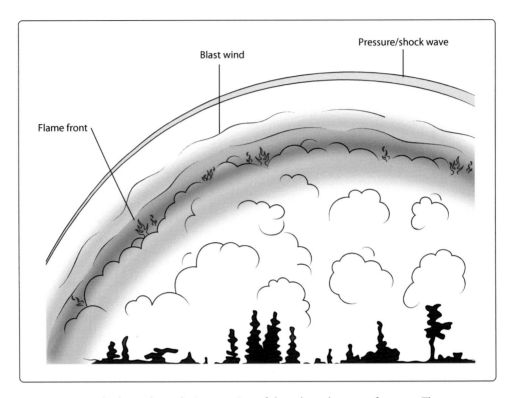

Figure 2.15 A high-grade explosion consists of three broad waves of energy. The pressure or **shock wave** is a very high initial wave of pressure (within milliseconds) with heating of the surrounding atmosphere. The second is the **blast wind** leading to mass air movements in the form of wind. It has a lower velocity compared to the initial shock wave, but may carry gas and debris further than the shock wave. Finally, there is the **flame front** after ignition of the surrounding environment.

affect is reflected in human tissue in the lungs, whereby the blast wave travelling through relatively incompressible blood disrupts the endothelium of the capillary wall as the wave enters the air-fluid interface of the alveolus.

Implosion
Implosion occurs when blood and air mix in the alveolus causing air emboli and bleeding leading to adult respiratory distress syndrome and acute lung injury (ALI).

Inertia
Inertial effects occur at the interface of tissue of different densities, with the lighter tissue being accelerated more than the heavier one, resulting in stress at the boundary.

Specific organ blast injuries

The ear
The tympanic membrane is the structure most frequently damaged in a primary blast injury. A sudden increase in pressure by as little as 5 psi above atmospheric pressure (1 atm is equivalent to 14.7 psi or 760 mmHg) will rupture the human eardrum, manifested by

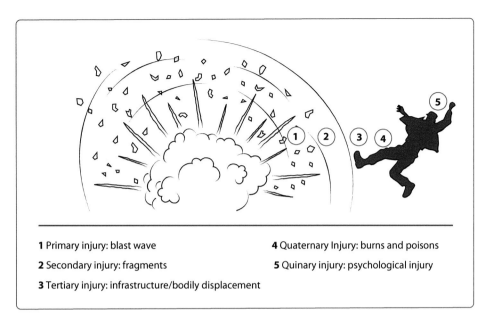

1 Primary injury: blast wave

2 Secondary injury: fragments

3 Tertiary injury: infrastructure/bodily displacement

4 Quaternary Injury: burns and poisons

5 Quinary injury: psychological injury

Figure 2.16 Blast injury classification.

deafness, tinnitus and vertigo. At higher dynamic pressures the bones within the middle ear may dislocate with traumatic disruption of the oval or round windows leading to permanent hearing loss (In the aftermath of the 2004 Madrid bombing, ruptured tympanic membranes were reported in in 99 of 243 victims).

The lung
The lung is the second most susceptible organ to primary blast injury. Pressure differentials across the alveolar/capillary interface lead to disruption, haemorrhage, contusion, pneumothorax, haemothorax, pneumomediastinum and subcutaneous emphysema. Chest x-ray (CXR) findings include a butterfly pattern similar to severe acute respiratory distress syndrome (ARDS) and referred to as 'blast lung'. These injuries are life threatening whose manifestations may be delayed depending on severity, but acute-onset pulmonary oedema is associated with a poor prognosis. Systemic acute air embolism (alveolar disruption) may affect cerebral and spinal cord vasculature, separate from any direct neurological traumatic injury or concussion. Typically, 40% of deaths after a blast injury are due to pulmonary complications of which 50% present acutely and a further 50% delayed (12–24 hours).

Hollow viscus organs
Rupture of the colon and less frequently, the small intestine may occur acutely (from the blast wave) or delayed (mesenteric ischaemia from vessel thrombosis).

Solid organs
When very high forces are involved, rupture of solid organs (e.g. liver, spleen, kidney) may occur, but more typically there is contusion, haemorrhage and ischaemia of the

tissue. In addition, abdominal injury is more common with underwater and closed space explosions, due to the higher or prolonged overpressure effects.

Secondary blast injury

Secondary blast injuries occur from energised debris, leading to a combination of blunt and penetrating injuries. Penetrating injuries may include primary fragments from the weapon itself (i.e. shrapnel) and/or secondary fragments (debris taking flight from the explosion) and are the leading cause of death after major building collapse, including asphyxiation, hypoxia and chest compression. Crush syndrome may also occur after structural collapse and entrapment, leading to metabolic derangement from extensive muscle tissue damage with subsequent release of myoglobin, urates, potassium and phosphates leading to hyperkalaemia, compartment syndrome and renal failure (toxic myoglobinuria).

Compartment syndrome after crushing results from compression of damaged, oedematous muscle within its inelastic fascial sheath, with swelling, which if left unreleased promotes local tissue ischaemia, which in turn enters a vicious cycle of increased swelling, increased compartment pressures, decreased tissue perfusion and further ischaemia/necrosis. Fasciotomy or compartment decompression should be performed as soon as it is safe to do so, with fluid resuscitation and treatment of the hyperkalaemia.

An estimated 1%-7% of injured patients after an explosion will suffer a traumatic amputation, from the high blast overpressure forces with bony fractures while concomitant strong blast winds rupture and strip away soft tissue structures leading to partial or complete extremity amputation. Traumatic amputation victims also have a very high mortality rate from other primary blast injuries, reflecting the magnitude of the blast.

The distance over which fragments may travel and cause injury is in fact much greater than the distance over which the blast overpressure typically travels. Thus, aerodynamic fragments may cause secondary injury hundreds or even thousands of metres remote from the explosion epicentre, whereas primary injury will typically occur within tens of metres of the epicentre (where its effect is greatest). Therefore, secondary blast injuries are more common than primary blast injuries, as they cover a greater area and distance affecting a greater number of casualties.

Tertiary blast injury

Tertiary blast injuries result from the forceful, physical displacement of a person by the force of the peak overpressure and/or blast wind leading to sustained blunt trauma (e.g. closed traumatic brain injury [TBI], blunt abdominal trauma, tissue contusions and bony fractures).

Quaternary and quinary blast injuries

Quaternary blast injuries include burns (chemical or thermal), toxic inhalation, exposure to radiation, asphyxiation (including carbon monoxide and cyanide after incomplete combustion of materials), and inhalation of dust containing carbon or asbestos. Dust inhalation was the commonest cause of death in Syria from barrel bombs. Burns are present in up to 30% of those injured by blast and are associated with increased mortality as inhalation increases the pulmonary damage. They are also complicated by crush injuries, making debridement difficult, compounded with high infection rates. Aggressive crystalloid resuscitation is crucial after thermal burns, although abdominal compartment syndrome and extremity myonecrosis occurs with excessive resuscitation. There is a recent addition to the nomenclature with quinary injuries used to categorise post traumatic stress disorder (PTSD) and other long term debilitating illnesses.

Treatment of blast injuries

General treatment

The approach to the victim is the same as any trauma with initial assessment and treatment of the immediate life-threatening injuries including airway, chest trauma management and haemorrhage control. We recommend aiming for a palpable radial pulse (approximates to about 90 mmHg) which will maintain adequate end-organ perfusion (e.g. cerebral mentation) at least temporarily, until the patient can be more adequately assessed in hospital with advanced or operative haemorrhage control as required.

Specific treatments

Crush injury

Intravenous fluid therapy is recommended to maintain renal perfusion and an adequate urine output (whilst avoiding fluid overload) to prevent (or treat) the toxic effects of myoglobinuria.

Ears

Once immediate life support measures have been instituted or life-threatening injuries ruled out, check for eardrum perforation with auroscopy (otoscopy). In addition to diagnosing injury to the ear, otoscopy is a good triage tool. If the tympanic membranes are intact, then the likelihood of severe primary blast injury may be reasonably excluded in the absence of other associated symptoms (e.g. dyspnoea, respiratory distress, abdominal pain).

Lung injury

If, however, the tympanic membranes are ruptured, patients should undergo CXR (most trauma patients will anyway) with observation for at least 8 hours (in the absence of other injuries requiring treatment) or as clinically indicated. As previously stated, blast injuries can be insidious with a delayed onset. Patients should have oxygen saturations monitored closely (pulse oximetry) or even intermittent CXR. A low PaO_2 or $\%SatO_2$ will signal early blast lung. The treatment of blast lung is typically supportive, with maintenance of oxygenation and ventilation as required. Rarely extracorporeal membrane oxygenation (ECMO) may be required, but this is associated with a very high mortality as it reflects the magnitude of the initial blast pressure.

Other organs

About 10% of patients will have ocular trauma ranging from rupture of the globe, hyphema and conjunctival haemorrhage. Cardiac blast injury described in the literature includes cardiac contusion, myocardial wall haemorrhage and atrial rupture. Finally, TBI may occur, ranging from severe diffuse axonal injury (primary), direct head trauma with blunt or penetrating effects (secondary), or milder cases including mild TBI and concussion.

Landmine injuries

Landmines may be triggered by a number of mechanisms including pressure, movement, sound, magnetism and vibration. Mines may also produce injuries when picked up accidentally resulting in hand and/or distal forearm traumatic amputation. When a landmine is stepped upon, the localised blast wave is directed upwards leading to a fragmentation injury (**Figure 2.17**). As the mine is typically under shallow ground, the fragmentation effects are comprised of both shrapnel from the mine and mud/dirt from the ground itself. This fragmentation injury is similar to ballistic injury, dependent on the amount of explosive and energy deposited.

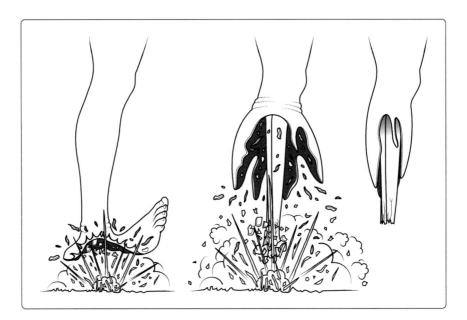

Figure 2.17 Stepping on a mine: There is an umbrella-like effect as the blast travels upwards from the ground, and damage occurs to the muscles of the lower leg. Typically, the foot is blown away and the blast wind strips the muscle from the bones of the limb. Fragmentation represents the dirt and mud forced upwards from the ground into muscle and soft tissues in the remainder of the limb. Managing this injury is both time-consuming and labour intensive on a service. Initially, a social scrub may be used with copious amounts of betadine/soap and water to remove gross contamination. Non-viable muscle is sharply debrided back to viable tissue (i.e. tissue actively bleeds with visible muscle contractions on stimulation). The wound may then be dressed and packed with gauze with a planned relook in the operating theatre 2–3 days later where further debridement of non-viable tissue is performed (i.e. soft tissue necrosis is dynamic) or the dressings changed and the bone of the lower leg amputated (typically a below knee amputation around day 5–6).

Additional reading

Aboudara M, Hicks B, Cuadrado D, Mahoney PF, Docekal J. Letter to the Editor: Impact of primary blast lung injury during combat operations in Afghanistan. *J R Army Med Corps* 2015. doi:10.1136/jramc-2015-000481.

Aboudara M, Mahoney PF, Hicks B, Cuadrado D. Primary blast lung injury at a NATO Role 3 hospital. *J R Army Med Corps* 2014;160(2):161–166.

Akhaddar A, Abouchadi A, Jidal M et al. Metallic foreign body in the sphenoid sinus after ballistic injury: A case report. *J Neuroradiol* 2008;35(2):125–128.

Argyros GJ. Management of primary blast injury. *Toxicology* 1997;121(1):105–115.

Avidan V, Hersch M, Armon Y et al. Blast lung injury: Clinical manifestations, treatment, and outcome. *Am J Surg* 2005;190(6):927–931.

Bowley DM, Gillingham S, Mercer S, Schrager JJ, West A. Pneumoperitoneum without visceral trauma: An under-recognised phenomenon after blast injury? *J R Army Med Corps* 2013;159(4):312–313.

Breeze J, Allanson-Bailey LS, Hepper AE, Midwinter MJ. Demonstrating the effectiveness of body armour: A pilot prospective computerised surface wound mapping trial performed at the Role 3 hospital in Afghanistan. *J R Army Med Corps* 2015;161(1):36–41.

Breeze J, Fryer R, Lewis EA, Clasper J. Defining the minimum anatomical coverage required to protect the axilla and arm against penetrating ballistic projectiles. *J R Army Med Corps* 2016;162(4):270–275.

Breeze J, Lewis EA, Fryer R, Hepper AE, Mahoney PF, Clasper JC. Defining the essential anatomical coverage provided by military body armour against high energy projectiles. *J R Army Med Corps* 2016;162(4):284–290.

Brogden TG, Garner JP. Anorectal injury in pelvic blast. *J R Army Med Corps* 2013;159(Suppl 1):i26–i31.

Carroll AW, Soderstrom CA. A new nonpenetrating ballistic injury. *Ann Surg* 1978;188(6):753–757.

Chen Y, Huang W, Constantini S. Concepts and strategies for clinical management of blast-induced traumatic brain injury and posttraumatic stress disorder. *J Neuropsychiatry Clin Neurosci* 2013;25(2):103–110.

Cherney LR, Gardner P, Logemann JA et al. Communication Sciences, and Disorders Clinical Trails Research Group. The role of speech-language pathology and audiology in the optimal management of the service member returning from Iraq or Afghanistan with a blast-related head injury: Position of the Communication Sciences and Disorders Clinical Trials Research Group. *J Head Trauma Rehabil* 2010;25(3):219–224.

Coley E, Roach P, Macmillan AI, West AT, Johnston AM. Penetrating paediatric thoracic injury. *J R Army Med Corps* 2011;157(3):243–245.

Cooper BR, Mellor A, Bruce A, Hall A, Mahoney PF. Paediatric thoracic damage control resuscitation for ballistic injury: A case report. *J R Army Med Corps* 2007;153(4):317–318.

Durrant JJ, Ramasamy A, Salmon MS, Watkin N, Sargeant I. Pelvic fracture-related urethral and bladder injury. *J R Army Med Corps* 2013;159(Suppl 1):i32–i39.

Eardley WG, Beaven A, Sargeant I. Endoscopic evaluation of a complex ballistic injury. *J R Army Med Corps* 2011;157(4):399–401.

Fries CA, Penn-Barwell J, Tai NR, Hodgetts TJ, Midwinter MJ, Bowley DM. Management of intestinal injury in deployed UK hospitals. *J R Army Med Corps* 2011;157(4):370–373.

Garth RJ. Blast injury of the ear: An overview and guide to management. *Injury* 1995;26(6):363–366.

Goh SH. Bomb blast mass casualty incidents: Initial triage and management of injuries. *Singapore Med J* 2009;50(1):101–106.

Guzzi LM, Argyros G. The management of blast injury. *Eur J Emerg Med* 1996;3(4):252–355.

Hare SS, Goddard I, Ward P, Naraghi A, Dick EA. The radiological management of bomb blast injury. *Clin Radiol* 2007;62(1):1–9.

Herry Y, Boucher F, Neyret P, Ferry T, Lustig S. Three-step sequential management for knee arthroplasty after severe ballistic injury: Two cases. *Orthop Traumatol Surg Res* 2016;102(1):131–134.

Jansen JO, Thomas GO, Adams SA et al. Early management of proximal traumatic lower extremity amputation and pelvic injury caused by improvised explosive devices (IEDs). *Injury* 2012;43(7):976–979.

Johnson D, Cartagena CM, Tortella FC, Dave JR, Schmid KE, Boutte AM. Acute and sub-acute microRNA dysregulation is associated with cytokine responses in the rodent model of penetrating ballistic-like brain injury. *J Trauma Acute Care Surg* 2017;83(Suppl 1):S145–S149.

Kumar V, Singh AK, Kumar P et al. Blast injury face: An exemplified review of management. *Natl J Maxillofac Surg* 2013;4(1):33–39.

LaCombe DM, Miller GT, Dennis JD. Primary blast injury: An EMS guide to pathophysiology, assessment & management. *JEMS* 2004;29(5):70–72, 74, 76–78, 80–81, 86–89.

Lavery GG, Lowry KG. Management of blast injuries and shock lung. *Curr Opin Anaesthesiol* 2004;17(2):151–157.

Ling G, Ecklund JM, Bandak FA. Brain injury from explosive blast: Description and clinical management. *Handb Clin Neurol* 2015;127:173–180.

Mackenzie IM, Tunnicliffe B. Blast injuries to the lung: Epidemiology and management. *Philos Trans R Soc Lond B Biol Sci* 2011;366(1562):295–299.

Mellor SG. The pathogenesis of blast injury and its management. *Br J Hosp Med* 1988;39(6):536–539.

Morrison JJ, Clasper JC, Gibb I, Midwinter M. Management of penetrating abdominal trauma in the conflict environment: The role of computed tomography scanning. *World J Surg* 2011;35(1):27–33.

Morrison JJ, Dickson EJ, Jansen JO, Midwinter MJ. Utility of admission physiology in the surgical triage of isolated ballistic battlefield torso trauma. *J Emerg Trauma Shock* 2012;5(3):233–2337.

Morrison JJ, Hunt N, Midwinter M, Jansen J. Associated injuries in casualties with traumatic lower extremity amputations caused by improvised explosive devices. *Br J Surg* 2012;99(3):362–366.

Morrison JJ, Mellor A, Midwinter M, Mahoney PF, Clasper JC. Is pre-hospital thoracotomy necessary in the military environment? *Injury* 2011;42(5):469–473.

Morrison JJ, Midwinter MJ, Jansen JO. Ballistic thoracoabdominal injury: Analysis of recent military experience in Afghanistan. *World J Surg* 2011;35(6):1396–1401.

Morrison JJ, Poon H, Garner J, Midwinter MJ, Jansen JO. Nontherapeutic laparotomy in combat casualties. *J Trauma Acute Care Surg* 2012;73(6 Suppl 5):S479–S482.

Mossadegh S, Tai N, Midwinter M, Parker P. Improvised explosive device related pelvi-perineal trauma: Anatomic injuries and surgical management. *J Trauma Acute Care Surg* 2012;73(2 Suppl 1):S24–S31.

Murakami Y, Wei G, Yang X et al. Brain oxygen tension monitoring following penetrating ballistic-like brain injury in rats. *J Neurosci Methods* 2012;203(1):115–121.

Mutafchiiski V, Popivanov G. Damage control surgery and open abdomen in trauma patients with exsanguinating bleeding. *Khirurgiia (Sofiia)* 2014;(1):4–10.

Pizov R, Oppenheim-Eden A, Matot I et al. Blast lung injury from an explosion on a civilian bus. *Chest* 1999;115(1):165–172.

Polzer H, Mutschler W. [Vacuum assisted closure therapy. Management of a severe blast injury to the lower limb]. *Unfallchirurg* 2012;115(9):792–797.

Quinones PM, Mentzer C, White C, Abuzeid A. Management of mangled extremity from shotgun blast injury. *Am Surg* 2016;82(8):200–201.

Round JA, Mellor AJ. Anaesthetic and critical care management of thoracic injuries. *J R Army Med Corps* 2010;156(3):145–149.

Sasser SM, Sattin RW, Hunt RC, Krohmer J. Blast lung injury. *Prehosp Emerg Care* 2006;10(2):165–172.

Sharma DM, Bowley DM. Immediate surgical management of combat-related injury to the external genitalia. *J R Army Med Corps* 2013;159(Suppl 1):i18–i20.

Sims K, Montgomery HR, Dituro P, Kheirabadi BS, Butler FK. Management of external hemorrhage in tactical combat casualty care: The adjunctive use of XStat compressed hemostatic sponges: TCCC guidelines change 15-03. *J Spec Oper Med* 2016;16(1):19–28.

Smith IM, Beech ZK, Lundy JB, Bowley DM. A prospective observational study of abdominal injury management in contemporary military operations: Damage control laparotomy is associated with high survivability and low rates of fecal diversion. *Ann Surg* 2015;261(4):765–773.

Smith JE. Blast lung injury. *J R Nav Med Serv* 2011;97(3):99–105.

Smith JE. The epidemiology of blast lung injury during recent military conflicts: A retrospective database review of cases presenting to deployed military hospitals, 2003–2009. *Philos Trans R Soc Lond B Biol Sci* 2011;366(1562):291–294.

Smith JE, Midwinter M, Lambert AW. Avoiding cavity surgery in penetrating torso trauma: The role of the computed tomography scan. *Ann R Coll Surg Engl* 2010;92(6):486–488.

Turegano-Fuentes F, Perez-Diaz D, Sanz-Sanchez M, Alfici R, Ashkenazi I. Abdominal blast injuries: Different patterns, severity, management, and prognosis according to the main mechanism of injury. *Eur J Trauma Emerg Surg* 2014;40(4):451–460.

Uppal L, Anderson P, Evriviades D. Complex lower genitourinary reconstruction following combat-related injury. *J R Army Med Corps* 2013;159(Suppl 1):i49–i51.

Waid-Ebbs JK, BCBA-D, Daly J et al. Response to goal management training in veterans with blast-related mild traumatic brain injury. *J Rehabil Res Dev* 2014;51(10):1555–1566.

Williams G, O'Malley M. Surgical considerations in the management of combined radiation blast injury casualties caused by a radiological dirty bomb. *Injury* 2010;41(9):943–947.

Williams RJ, Fries CA, Midwinter M, Lambert AW. Battlefield scrotal trauma: How should it be managed in a deployed military hospital? *Injury* 2013;44(9):1246–1249.

Wood AM, Trimble K, Louden MA, Jansen J. Selective non-operative management of ballistic abdominal solid organ injury in the deployed military setting. *J R Army Med Corps* 2010;156(1):21–24.

Zhao GJ, Cheng JY, Zhi SC, Jin X, Lu ZQ. Conservative management of esophageal perforation due to external air-blast injury: A case report and literature review. *Therap Adv Gastroenterol* 2015;8(4):234–238.

3 | Emergency Surgical Airway

Morgan McMonagle

The *emergency surgical airway (ESA)* is a true emergency defined as *creation of an opening in the anterior airway through a non-anatomical route for the purposes of emergency oxygenation and ventilation.*

The clinical scenario is typically immediately life-threatening, often described as *'can't intubate–can't ventilate'* with an imminent threat to life. It is a true 'time-critical' procedure, as adequate oxygenation often cannot be maintained. The typical scenario in trauma is after a failed attempt at emergency crash intubation or emergency rapid sequence intubation (RSI) with the one or more of the following:

1. *Can't intubate*
2. *Can't ventilate*
3. *Failed attempt at intubation where immediate control of the airway is mandatory*
   Typically, this is a non-airway issue but where there is immediate need for surgery (i.e. predicted clinical course mandates immediate surgery), but there has been a failure to achieve a secure airway through conventional means (e.g. stab wound to chest with shock and need for trauma thoracotomy)

The trauma bay must always have ESA equipment present and ready for use, preferably in a separate, easily accessible kit. Conditions with a *predicted difficult airway* include; serious facial injuries, facial and airway burns, known airway difficulty pre-hospital, traumatic brain injury with trismus, laryngeal trauma or any other neck haematoma/swelling.

Predicted difficult airway

If time and circumstances allow, the airway team may predict on clinical examination that the patient has a higher probability than normal of having a 'difficult' airway for RSI and thus may on balance opt to use another airway (non-surgical) adjunct (i.e. a 'difficult' intubation may be predicted and steps taken to mitigate the risk). This is particularly important in trauma care, as, by definition all airway management is potentially difficult, especially when the C-spine requires immobilisation. However, in the trauma setting, a cuffed endotracheal (ET) tube is the *definitive* airway of choice. Video-assisted laryngoscopy has become the current standard of care for acute airway management in trauma, but the surgeon should be prepared to intervene with an ESA if RSI is either unsuccessful or not achievable in a timely manner.

Failed airway (can't intubate)

There is no one definition for a failed airway, but unsuccessful tracheal intubation after *three* attempts (in a timely and progressive manner) or an unrecognised failure to intubate the trachea (e.g. oesophageal intubation) where harm or potential harm has occurred are accepted as defining scenarios. In the early stages of managing the difficult airway, the technique of choice depends on whether O_2Sats can be maintained >94% with bag-mask ventilation (BMV) alone:

- **Can't intubate, but can ventilate (O_2Sats >94% with BMV)**
- **Can't intubate and can't ventilate (O_2Sats <94% despite BMV)**

Can't intubate but can ventilate (O_2Sats >94%)

Although there is a failure to achieve a definitive airway, the airway team can at least temporarily maintain O_2Sats >94% with BMV alone (one or two rescuer technique). A number of other *anaesthetic rescue airway techniques* may be employed (*Table 3.1*), but the trauma surgeon must be prepared to intervene if a definitive airway is not achieved.

Can't intubate and can't ventilate (O_2Sats <94%)

This is an absolute airway emergency! Intubation has been unsuccessful in parallel with failure to maintain O_2Sats adequately to maintain life. Any further attempts at standard

Table 3.1 Airway rescue techniques

Airway rescue techniques (O_2Sats >94% with BMV)		
First-line technique*	Bag mask ventilation (BMV)	Simplest technique for maintaining oxygenation and ventilation; can be operated by one or two rescuers
Surgical airway (O_2Sats <94% with BMV)		
Percutaneous	Needle cricothyroidotomy	May provide supplemental oxygenation, albeit short-lived and therefore its utility is of questionable value
	Percutaneous cricothyroidotomy	More steps involved and longer to perform compared with open cricothyroidotomy, therefore not the technique of choice
Open	Open surgical cricothyroidotomy	The technique of choice in the failed intubation after trauma with deteriorating patient
	Open tracheostomy	Difficult and takes too long to perform in an emergency setting; not recommended

* Although BMV is the first line technique to improve oxygenation after failed intubation, second line anaesthetic techniques in an attempt to obtain a secure airway may include; video-assisted laryngoscopy, fibreoptic-assisted intubation, light stylet intubation, laryngeal mask airway (LMA), intubating LMA and the combitube. A detailed description of these techniques and equipment is beyond the scope of this book.

intubation, even with non-surgical rescue techniques, will likely lead to uncontrolled and rapid further desaturation with immediate risk of cardiac arrest. Typically in trauma, there is an obstruction at the level of the larynx (e.g. haematoma, laryngeal fracture) or there has been an unrecognised oesophageal intubation (with further desaturation).

An emergency surgical airway is the rescue technique of choice!

Emergency surgical airway techniques

Four ESA techniques are described in textbooks:

1. Needle emergency cricothyroidotomy
2. Percutaneous emergency cricothyroidotomy
3. Open emergency cricothyroidotomy
4. Open emergency tracheostomy

For the purposes of acute trauma management, we advocate always using *open (surgical) cricothyroidotomy* as the 'go-to' technique of choice. An open cricothyroidotomy is the most rapidly effective and safest approach, thus establishing a definitive, protected airway, effectively managing both oxygenation and ventilation. The percutaneous and needle techniques are more time-consuming to perform and do not provide a protected (cuffed) airway in the trauma patient. In addition, they do not adequately oxygenate or ventilate the shocked patient. An open tracheostomy is difficult and cumbersome to perform as an emergency in addition to being too time-consuming. This is due to the position of the trachea in the neck and the overlying tissues. Although useful in the more controlled, elective setting, the trachea is a short structure that travels in an anterior-to-posterior direction before diving behind the inaccessible retrosternal space. In addition, the strap muscles and thyroid isthmus lie anterior on the trachea, notwithstanding any haematoma or other tissue trauma that may be present, will make this too challenging in the acute trauma setting.

An open (surgical) cricothyroidotomy is the technique of choice for ESA!

Open emergency cricothyroidotomy

Ideally, this should be performed under sterile conditions, but do not delay if sterilising solution is not readily available.

Anatomy and landmarks

The cricothyroid membrane (CTM) is the ideal access point to the airway. It resides in a superficial position along the anterior neck approximately midway between the sternal notch and the floor of the mouth (**Figures 3.1 and 3.2**). It is easily palpated (in health) lying between the cricoid and thyroid cartilages as a slight dip in the skin. It is just subcutaneous (little tissue to dissect through) and is a thin, easily perforated avascular membrane. However, be aware that in the trauma setting these anatomical landmarks may be distorted by a combination of tissue injury, swelling and/or the presence of haematoma.

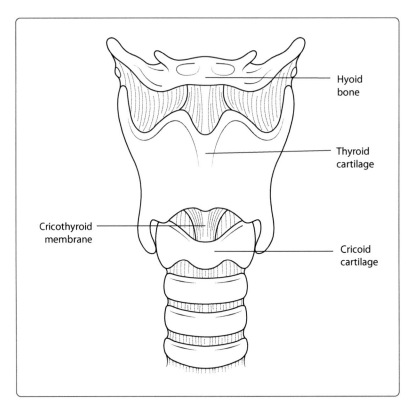

Figure 3.1 Anatomy for surgical airway. The cricothyroid membrane is the short ligament stretching from the cricoid cartilage (lowermost ring) to the thyroid cartilage (largest and most prominent structure) in the midline anterior neck and serves as the 'gatekeeper' for ESA. It lies superficial, only covered with skin and subcutaneous tissue and in health may be palpated as a slight 'dip' in the midline neck structures (this of course may be obscured by trauma, swelling or haematoma). It is an avascular plane allowing direct access to the airway without haemorrhage and below the vocal cords. All personnel managing trauma and / or the emergency airway should be familiar with this anatomy and the technique of performing a cricothyroidotomy.

Position and preparation

The patient should be supine. If C-spine immobilisation is not required, surface anatomy recognition can be enhanced by using slight head-tilt (remove the pillow!) and even a small 'raise' or 'roll' behind the upper thorax (e.g. rolled up towel). However, this is typically an impractical step in the emergency trauma scenario. Local anaesthesia (with epinephrine) should be infiltrated in the awake patient (allows anaesthesia of the skin with reduced bleeding), best infiltrated on either side of the CTM (to avoid distorting the anatomy in the mid-line).

The tracheostomy tube and equipment should have been checked beforehand (i.e. balloon inflation). A gum elastic bougie (the type used in regular RSI) is a useful adjunct which may be inserted into the airway first before railroading the tracheostomy tube over it and into position. Ventilation equipment and tubing must also be available, in addition to monitoring equipment (O_2 saturations and end-tidal CO_2 monitoring are mandatory).

The incision

A *longitudinal* (not transverse!) incision is made in the midline of the neck to maximise the chance of successful exposure of the CTM quickly and safely (**Figures 3.2 and 3.3**). Use a long incision, as cosmesis is not important. Try to centre the incision over the anterior airway structures in case of distortion secondary to trauma. Transverse incisions run the

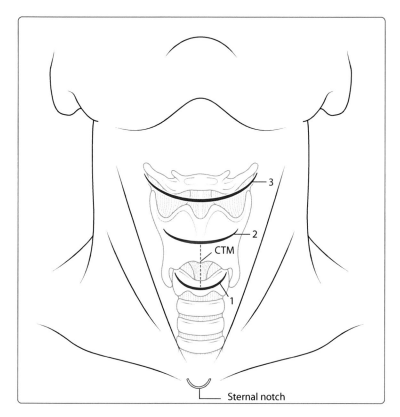

Figure 3.2 Surface anatomy for emergency open cricothyroidotomy. Surface anatomy consists of the cricoid cartilage (1: lower most midline ring), thyroid cartilage (2: largest and most prominent midline cartilage) and the hyoid bone (3). The CTM is an avascular, superficial midline ligament stretching from the cricoid cartilage to the thyroid cartilage, lying just below skin and subcutaneous tissue. It is often palpable as a slight 'dip' in the midline neck. A longitudinal incision is the best approach to expose the CTM. If a transverse incision is created (under the pressure of an emergency airway scenario), there is a risk of creating an incision at the incorrect level, thereby missing the CTM and prolonging the time during which the patient is starved of oxygen. In addition, there are ergonomic advantages to this approach, whereby the surgeon can steady the mid-neck airway complex with his/her left hand, whilst using the surgical blade in his/her right hand to create the longitudinal surgical incision.

Important surface anatomy

- Sternal notch
- Cricoid bone
- Thyroid cartilage
- The cricothyroid membrane (CTM)
  - Soft 'dip' between the cricoid bone and thyroid cartilage in the midline of anterior neck

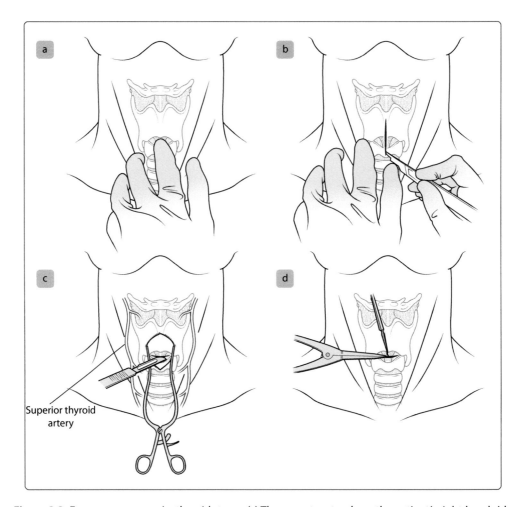

Figure 3.3 Emergency open cricothyroidotomy. (a) The operator stands on the patient's right-hand side and grips the thyroid cartilage using the left hand. This holds the midline structures in position, whilst the index finger slides inferiorly into the 'dip' of the CTM. (b) The left-hand grip maintains the airway structures in position. Taking a surgical scalpel (10 or 15 blade) in the right hand, a longitudinal (not transverse) incision in the skin and subcutaneous tissues is made from the thyroid cartilage to just below the cricoid ring. (c) The CTM is identified and an incision (typically transverse below the skin incision) is made to gain access to the airway. Care must be taken to always remain within the midline, so as to avoid injuring the superior thyroid vessels and causing bleeding. Upon piercing the CTM, air may be felt and heard exhaled form the lungs. (d) If available, a tracheostomy hook may be used to elevate the thyroid cartilage and a tracheal dilator used to widen the opening to the CTM. If not available, the upturned handle of the surgical blade may be inserted and twisted to widen the opening.

risk of being located at the wrong level, thereby missing the CTM, thereby requiring an additional incision(s), whilst time rapidly slips by. However, by using a sizable longitudinal incision, the chances of successful and rapid exposure of the CTM are much greater.

Further steps

Once a long longitudinal, midline incision is made between the cricoid cartilage and thyroid cartilage, the CTM will quickly come into view. With extensive tissue injury

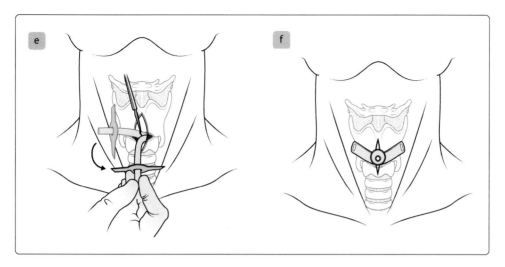

Figure 3.3 (Continued) (e) The pre-checked tracheostomy tube is inserted using a slight twisting motion into the trachea. If in doubt, use a size 6 tube. If not available, a regular ET tube may be inserted and the balloon inflated. (f) The airway tube comes to rest within the airway and should be sutured to the skin to hold in place. Its correct position within the airway must be checked the same as post-RSI, especially with evidence of $ETCO_2$.

or bleeding, the CTM may be palpated rather than seen. Once exposed, open the CTM (transverse or longitudinal) with the surgical knife. The handle of the scalpel may then be inserted and rotated to widen the CTM opening or, if available, a tracheal dilator inserted for the same effect. The tracheostomy tube (typically 6.0–6.5 size) is then inserted in a caudal direction into the airway and the balloon inflated to create an effective airway seal, rendering it 'protected'. Only inflate enough air into the pilot balloon cuff to generate an effective seal (although in the emergency situation this is less important as the cuff pressure may be checked later and the pressure managed accordingly). If a tracheostomy tube is not available, use a regular endotracheal (ET) tube, remembering that it is longer and therefore more vulnerable to dislodgement.

Why is emergency open tracheostomy not recommended?

- Tracheal anatomy is difficult to appreciate in an emergency
  - Short passage in the neck
  - Passes superiorly to inferior and slightly posteriorly as it travels into the chest
  - Inaccessible in the chest
- The anatomy is difficult to palpate, unless the patient is positioned correctly
  - Often not possible if cervical spine injury is suspected
- The trachea is often mobile and difficult to stabilise adequately
- An emergency tracheostomy takes too long to perform
  - Potentially starve the brain of O_2 for too long
- It is a more difficult technique to master
  - Not suitable in the emergency setting
- It requires adequate equipment
  - Lighting
  - Specialised equipment
  - Suture material for haemostasis

Post-insertion management

Once inserted, 'proof of placement' (i.e. within the airway) is mandatory which includes visualising end-tidal CO_2 (colour change capnogram or preferably visualising a CO_2 trace on the capnography monitor). In addition, there should be continuous O_2 saturation monitoring during and after the procedure.

Complications

The most important complication is failure to achieve the airway or failure to intervene on time leading to severe hypoxia, brain injury and/or cardiac arrest. Additional complications include pneumothorax, haemorrhage, haemorrhage into the airway with hypoxia, uncontrolled opening of a haematoma (especially arterial), airway trauma, posterior airway trauma with injury to the hypopharynx or oesophagus and injury to the carotid (if incision not kept midline).

A special note on isolated laryngeal trauma

This is one of the most challenging airway scenarios in trauma as there is a real risk of converting a partial upper airway obstruction (e.g. fractured larynx with partial impingement on the lumen) in the awake, self-ventilating patient into a complete airway obstruction (intubation of the false passage) with rapid hypoxaemia.

If awake and talking, allow the patient to temporarily protect their own airway and pre-oxygenate for >10 min. Preferably advanced airway management should take place in the operating room (in the absence of other competing trauma injuries) and the technique of choice is to perform an awake, fibre-optic intubation with inhalation anaesthesia if these skills are available. This technique involves the patient inhaling anaesthetic gas just enough to become sedated, perhaps augmented with low-dose IV sedation and local anaesthetic applied *via* droplet spray to the mouth and upper airway.

In addition, the anterior surface anatomy should be marked (especially CTM) in case open cricothyroidotomy becomes necessary and local anaesthetic injected appropriately prior to attempted intubation, in case of sudden deterioration or the development of a 'can't intubate–can't ventilate' scenario. If successful fibre-optic intubation is possible, then this should proceed safely. If complete obstruction or deterioration occurs, then a surgical airway (as described) is performed.

Additional reading

Bair AE, Filbin MR, Kilkarni RG et al. The failed intubation attempt in the emergency department: Analysis of prevalence, rescue techniques and personnel. *J Emerg Med* 2002;23:131–140.

Bair AE, Panacek EA, Wisner DH, Bales R, Sakles JC. Cricothyrotomy: A 5-year experience at one institution. *J Emerg Med* 2003;24(2):151–156.

Brofeldt BT, Panacek EA, Richards JR. An easy cricothyrotomy approach: The rapid four-step technique. *Acad Emerg Med* 1996;3(11):1060–1063.

Dunham CM, Barraco RD, Clark DE et al. Guidelines or emergency tracheal intubation immediately after traumatic injury. *J Trauma* 2003;55:162–179.

Erlandson MJ, Clinton JE, Ruiz E, Cohen J. Cricothyrotomy in the emergency department revisited. *J Emerg Med* 1989;7(2):115–118.

Fortune JB, Judkins DG, Scanzaroli D, McLeod KB, Johnson SB. Efficacy of prehospital surgical cricothyrotomy in trauma patients. *J Trauma* 1997;42(5):832–836; discussion 837–838.

Gens DR. Surgical airway management. In Tintinalli JE, Kelen GD, Stapczynski JS, eds. *Tintinalli's Emergency Medicine: A Comprehensive Study Guide*, 6th ed. New York: McGraw-Hill Companies, 2004.

Holcroft JW, Anderson JT, Sena MJ. Shock and acute pulmonary failure in surgical patients. In Doherty GM, ed. *Current Diagnosis & Treatment: Surgery*, 13th ed. New York: McGraw-Hill Companies, 2010:151–175.

Holmes JF, Panacek EA, Sakles JC, Brofeldt BT. Comparison of 2 cricothyrotomy techniques: Standard method versus rapid 4-step technique. *Ann Emerg Med* 1998 Oct;32(4):442–446.

Jacobson LE, Gomez GA, Sobieray RJ, Rodman GH, Solotkin KC, Misinski ME. Surgical cricothyroidotomy in trauma patients: Analysis of its use by paramedics in the field. *J Trauma* 1996;41(1):15–20.

Marx JA, Hockberger RS, Walls RM. Airway. In *Rosen's Emergency Medicine: Concepts and Clinical Practice*, vol. 1, 6th ed. Philadelphia: Mosby Elsevier, 2006.

McGill J, Clinton JE, Ruiz E. Cricothyrotomy in the emergency department. *Ann Emerg Med* 1982;11(7):361–364.

Miklus RM, Elliott C, Snow N. Surgical cricothyrotomy in the field: Experience of a helicopter transport team. *J Trauma* 1989;29(4):506–508.

Roberts H. Surgical cricothyrotomy. In *Clinical Procedures in Emergency Medicine*, 5th ed. Philadelphia: Saunders Elsevier, 2010.

Robinson KJ, Katz R, Jacobs LM. A 12-year experience with prehospital cricothyrotomies. *Air Med J* 2001;20(6): 27–30.

Sagarin MJ, Barton ED, Chng YM, Walls RM. Airway management by US and Canadian emergency medicine residents: A multicenter analysis of more than 6,000 endotracheal intubation attempts. *Ann Emerg Med* 2005;46(4):328–336.

Salvino CK, Dries D, Gamelli R et al. Emergency cricothyroidotomy in trauma victims. *J Trauma* 1993;34:503–505.

Spaite DW, Joseph M. Prehospital cricothyrotomy: An investigation of indications, technique, complications, and patient outcome. *Ann Emerg Med* 1990;19(3):279–285.

Strange GR, Niederman LG, Henretig FM, King C. Surgical cricothyrotomy. In *Textbook of Pediatric Emergency Procedures*. Baltimore: Williams & Wilkins, 1997: 351.

Talving P, Gelbard R. Cricothyroidotomy. In Demetriades D, Inaba K, Velmahos G, eds. *Atlas of Surgical Techniques in Trauma*. Cambridge: Cambridge University Press, 2015: *5–11*.

Toschlog EA, Sagraves SG, Rotondo MF. Airway control. In Feliciano DV, Mattox KL, Moore EE, eds. *Trauma*, 6th ed. New York: McGraw-Hill Companies, 2008: chap. 12.

Vissers RJ, Bair AE. Surgical airway management. In Walls RM, Murphy MF, eds. *Manual of Emergency Airway Management*, 4th ed. Philadelphia, PA: Lippincott Williams & Wilkins, 2012; chap. 18.

Wright MJ, Greenberg DE, Hunt JP et al. Surgical cricothyroidotomy in trauma patients. *South Med J* 2003;96:465–467.

4 Thoracic Surgery

James V. O'Connor

Introduction

Chest trauma is common, placed within the top three causes of death after injury but the second leading cause of death for those patients dying within one hour of hospital arrival (central nervous system injury being the premier cause). Despite this, approximately three-quarters of chest injuries may be successfully managed non-operatively with simple procedures such as chest drainage, chest physiotherapy and analgesia as appropriate. Those patients requiring surgery may have injuries ranging from minimal (intercostal vessel bleed) to catastrophic (great vessel rupture). For penetrating trauma, the conventional indications for exploration include:

- Any isolated thoracic injury with shock
- Initial chest tube output >1500 mL (some use 1000 mL)
- A persistent chest tube output >200 to 300 mL per hour over 3–4 hours
- Cardiac tamponade
- Massive air leak (with impaired oxygenation / ventilation)

The operative mortality following emergent thoracic exploration for trauma is variable but, in general, is reported to be about 30%. One large, multi-institutional study of traumatic lung injury reported a linear increase in operative mortality with the extent of pulmonary resection – tractotomy 13%, wedge resection 30%, lobectomy 43% and pneumonectomy 50% – which is generally consistent across the literature.

Analysis of outcomes following cardiac injury is challenging for several reasons, as many patients die in the field and the survival for those *in extremis* requiring a trauma bay thoracotomy remains low, with many studies combining both blunt and penetrating cohorts in the analysis. The reported mortality rates for patients after penetrating cardiac trauma alive on arrival at hospital is about 33%. A higher mortality is seen after gunshot injury, those requiring a trauma bay thoracotomy, low cardiovascular-respiratory scores on arrival or a cardiac rhythm on arrival other than sinus rhythm. Other studies have concluded cardiac tamponade to be protective (possibly different physiology), while others have not. Precordial penetrating injuries are especially worrisome and a cardiac injury must be excluded by ultrasound imaging, pericardial window or surgical exploration.

Tracheobronchial and oesophageal injuries

Tracheobronchial and oesophageal injuries are uncommon, but when present, are more prevalent in the neck compared with the true thorax, and may result from either blunt or penetrating injury. Compromise or loss of the airway is a dreaded complication with the potential for rapidly fatal consequences. Promptly (or pre-emptively) securing the airway requires sound judgment and advanced airway skills. Because these injuries are infrequent and most published series include both blunt and penetrating injuries, in addition to grouping both cervical and thoracic injured groups, outcomes are difficult to interpret. But, even with the inherent limitations of these studies several key principles can be formulated:

- Penetrating injuries occur more commonly in the neck and are often diagnosed on physical examination alone
- Conversely, blunt airway injuries are more commonly intra-thoracic with almost two-thirds occurring proximal to the carina
- A continuous air leak or a large persistent pneumothorax following tube thoracostomy should prompt further investigation (bronchoscopy is the modality of choice)

In general, tracheobronchial injuries require operative repair, and delayed repair is associated with a higher mortality and morbidity. The operative mortality for all tracheobronchial injuries is between 15% and 19%. Similarly, oesophageal injuries are uncommon and almost universally the result of penetrating trauma. Cervical oesophageal injury is more easily diagnosed and treated with a much lower morbidity and mortality. An intra-thoracic oesophageal injury is decidedly more difficult to diagnose and treat. A missed intra-thoracic oesophageal injury results in mediastinitis, sepsis and shock and carries a very high mortality. Mediastinal air seen on plain radiograph or CT requires further investigation. Oesophagoscopy and oesophagraphy are equally good at diagnosing oesophageal injury, but a combination of both modalities has a very high sensitivity and specificity. Operative mortality varies between 6% and 19%, but increases dramatically with delay in surgical intervention. Because of the high mortality associated with a delay in definitive treatment, it is imperative that the clinician rapidly excludes these injuries if suspected and if diagnosed, then a prompt, definitive operation is required.

Great vessel injuries

Great vessel injuries (aorta, aortic arch and its great branches) are daunting to manage. Life-threatening haemorrhage, challenging surgical exposure and a lack of experience treating these infrequent injuries all contribute to their lethality. Over half of patients die prior to reaching hospital with operative mortality rates up to 40%. Other associated adverse effects on outcomes include:

- Longer transport times
- Degree of shock on arrival
- Combined great vessel arterial and venous injuries

Rapid evaluation of patients presenting in shock is imperative. Physical examination should concentrate on cardiorespiratory status with an upper extremity neurovascular evaluation. A FAST scan, with both abdominal and pericardial views, and a portable chest x-ray complete the evaluation. Large bore central access should be placed in the femoral veins since thoracic great veins may be injured. Exposure is best obtained *via* a median sternotomy or clamshell thoracotomy. Haemodynamically stable patients may benefit from computer tomography angiography (CTA), which will change the surgical approach in 25% of cases. It needs to be emphasised that additional imaging (CTA, angio, duplex) is only appropriate in haemodynamically well patients in whom a great vessel injury is only suspected. With the exception of the superior vena cava (SVC) and inferior vena cava (IVC), the great veins in the chest may be ligated if injured. Arterial injuries are repaired with primary anastomosis (if tension-free) or with interposition grafting, with ligation reserved only for those *in extremis* if shunting is not feasible.

Thoracic injury damage control

A fundamental question the attending surgeon must address when operating for thoracic trauma is the role of *damage control*, which has demonstrated a survival benefit. The principles of damage control were first described for penetrating abdominal trauma (Chapter 1) and include:

- Rapid control of haemorrhage and contamination
- Resuscitation in the intensive care unit (with blood and blood products)
- Planned, definitive surgery once normal physiology is restored

These principles have also been successfully applied in vascular and orthopaedic trauma and more recently in damage control thoracic surgery. The decision to use damage control in managing thoracic injuries follow a few guiding considerations:

- Overall injury severity burden
- Thoracic injury severity burden
- Degree of coagulopathy
- Hypothermia
- Degree of acidosis (reflects depth of shock)
- The need for concomitant surgery (e.g. laparotomy, orthopaedic, extremity vascular)

The surgeon must carefully weigh these factors and exercise astute, sophisticated judgement. Rapid control of lung *parenchymal haemorrhage* is achieved using a stapler and often multiple loads are necessary to perform a non-anatomic resection for haemorrhage control. As described earlier, large veins (except SVC and IVC) may be ligated if injured and arteries repaired or shunted (if damage control required). The pleural space is drained and packs may be placed on the raw pleural surface and a temporary closure used. Once normal physiology is restored (typically 2–3 days), the patient is returned to the operating room, the packs removed, the plural spaces irrigated and the chest formally closed. A number of points are worth emphasising:

- Packs adjacent to the heart and mediastinum should not be packed too tightly (i.e. risk of tamponade!)
- Posteriorly placed large bore chest drains are essential (blood collects posteriorly when lying supine!)

If done correctly and appropriately, damage control thoracic surgery should not contribute to additional cardiorespiratory compromise.

Left anterolateral thoracotomy

The left anterolateral thoracotomy can be performed rapidly and provides adequate exposure to the left pleural space, which may be further extended into a clamshell thoracotomy (bilateral anterolateral thoracotomy) for greater exposure of the mediastinum and right hemithorax. The major disadvantage of the left anterolateral approach is the limited exposure of the posterior chest structures, but is the most commonly used approach for a resuscitative thoracotomy (trauma bay) in patients presenting *in extremis*.

Several techniques can improve exposure. Placing a bump under the back to elevate the chest by 20–30 degrees and extending the ipsilateral arm out of the field affords better visualisation (**Figure 4.1**). Positioning the patient in this manner allows the incision to be carried further posteriorly (right down to the gurney/bed) allowing improved exposure of the left pleural space. The incision follows the inferior (outer) border of the *pectoralis major* muscle (or infra-mammary fold (breast) in women) which corresponds to the 5th intercostal space, just inferior to the nipple. Do not count ribs, as this wastes

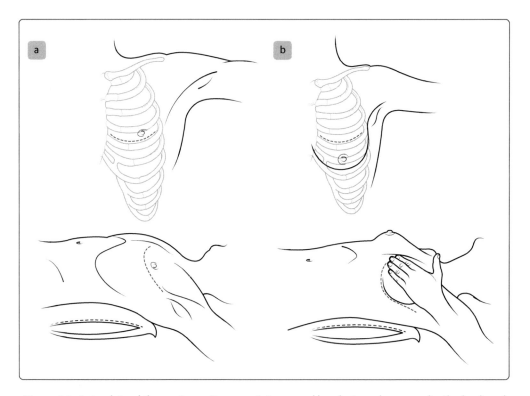

Figure 4.1 Anterolateral thoracotomy. Exposure is improved by placing a bump under the back and the fully extended ipsilateral arm. (a) The recommended position of the incision in the male patient following the outer (lateral) curve of the pectoralis muscle. (b) The recommended position of the incision in the female patient, which is generally identical, except that is follows the outer curve of the breast, which corresponds to the pectoralis muscle counterpart.

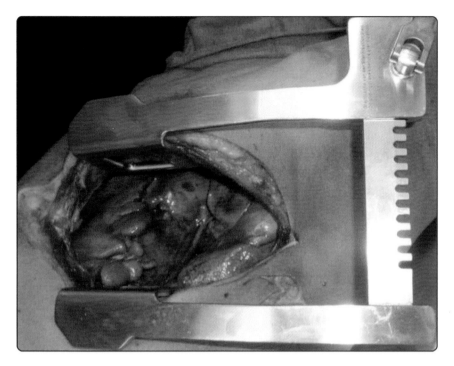

Figure 4.2 Chest exposure with a left anterolateral thoracotomy. The retractor's handle is positioned towards the axilla to facilitate extending the incision to a clamshell thoracotomy (if required).

time, causes confusion you will only get it wrong!. The incision starts at the left sternal border, follows the curve of the rib and extends as far posteriorly as possible. The 5th intercostal muscle is incised along the superior border of the rib below the space, avoiding the intercostal bundle on the upper rib's inferior surface. A Finochietto chest retractor is positioned with the handle *towards the axilla*. This allows the incision to be extended into a clamshell thoracotomy (if required), without needing to reposition the retractor. With the retractor widely opened the heart and left pleural space are easily accessed (**Figure 4.2**). Incising the inferior pulmonary ligament (fused parietal and visceral pleura) will mobilise the lung.

The pericardium is opened anterior (stay high on the heart) along its surface and parallel to the phrenic nerve in a longitudinal fashion (**Figure 4.3**). The heart is then delivered out of the pericardium (make sure the pericardial opening is large enough) and open cardiac massage may be performed if necessary. If required, the descending thoracic aorta may be crossed clamped from this approach. This manoeuvre may be challenging, as the aorta is typically collapsed if hypotensive/hypovolaemic, making the aorta more challenging to find. Rapidly incise the inferior pulmonary ligament to improve exposure (taking care not to injure the vessels at the inferior part of the left hilum) and, if time permits, placing a nasogastric tube will assist in identifying and distinguishing the thoracic aorta from the oesophagus. The distal mediastinal pleura overlying the descending thoracic aorta must be opened and the aorta is then bluntly dissected allowing the operator's left hand to encircle it while the cross clamp is placed with the right (**Figure 4.4**). Take care not to

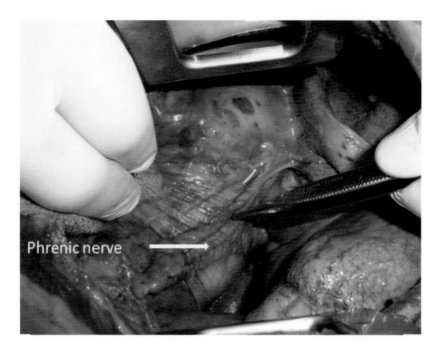

Figure 4.3 Pericardiotomy. The pericardium should be opened anterior and parallel to the phrenic nerve (arrow).

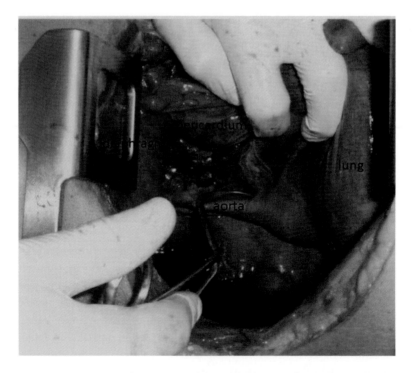

Figure 4.4 Aortic cross-clamping. To place an aortic cross clamp, the mediastinal pleura is bluntly dissected off the aorta (arrow) to allow complete occlusion. The cross clamp is placed achieving aortic occlusion. It is easy to misidentify the aorta in the hypotensive patient.

injure an intercostal branch, which will lead to additional bleeding. The pleura must be removed from the aorta (about 1–2 cm) to ensure effective cross-clamping of the correct structure and to prevent additional injury (especially intercostal branch avulsion).

Clamshell thoracotomy (bilateral anterolateral thoracotomy)

This incision affords superb access to the anterior mediastinum and both pleural spaces simultaneously, and is ideally suited as the resuscitative thoracotomy of choice. As mentioned earlier a left anterolateral thoracotomy can be extended into a clamshell. Using a Lebsche knife, sternal saw, trauma shears or bone cutters, the sternum is divided directly across horizontally. The incision is then extended as a right anterolateral 'mirror-image' thoracotomy (**Figure 4.5**). There are several key technical details:

- For maximum exposure, the incision must come across the body of the sternum (not the xiphoid!). There is a tendency to place the incision too inferiorly, which will seriously hamper exposure!
- The divided bilateral internal mammary arteries must be sought out and ligated, both proximally and distally, as they will bleed. In the profoundly hypotensive patient these vessels may not be appreciated immediately but still require ligation. If not ligated at the initial operation they will be when forced to re-explore for recurrent bleeding!

Fully opening bilateral rib spreaders yields excellent exposure to the anterior mediastinum and both hemithoraces (**Figure 4.6**). Almost all thoracic surgical procedures can be accomplished through this incision including pulmonary resection, cardiorrhaphy, great vessel and most tracheal repairs. There is, however, very limited exposure of posterior mediastinal structures.

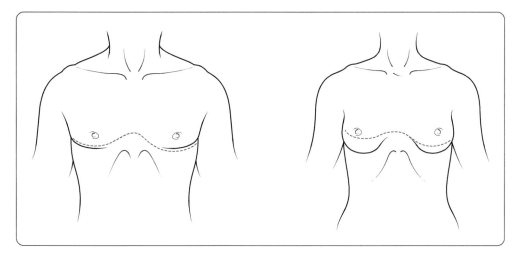

Figure 4.5 Clamshell thoracotomy. It is important to place the incision across the sternum, not the xiphoid. Placing the incision too inferiorly will hamper exposure. Some authorities advocate placing the right thoracic incision one intercostal space higher than the left for better access to the right hilum and aortic arch, but we prefer to keep the description simple as a mirror image incision, which is more than adequate.

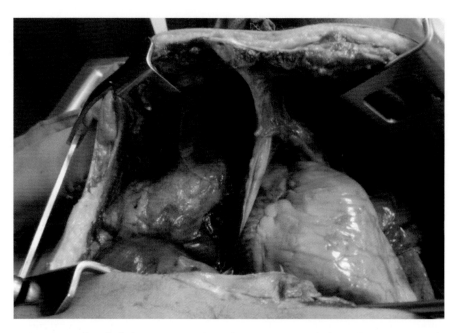

Figure 4.6 Clamshell thoracotomy. Bilateral retractors provided excellent exposure of both pleural spaces and the mediastinum.

Cardiac injuries

Cardiac injuries are suspected with any penetrating injury within the *cardiac box*, which is bounded superiorly by the clavicles, inferiorly by the costal margin and laterally by the midclavicular line (**Figure 4.7**). *The absence of hypotension does not exclude a possible cardiac injury* as the patient, especially if young, initially may be in compensated shock. The classic description of tamponade with Beck's triad (hypotension, distended neck veins and muffled

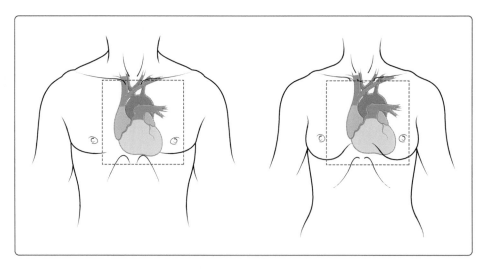

Figure 4.7 The cardiac box. The borders are inferior to the clavicles, superior to the costal margin and medial to both midclavicular lines. Penetrating injuries in this location must be evaluated for a potential cardiac injury.

heart sounds) is infrequently present and unreliable. A rapid bedside cardiac ultrasound exam is accurate, sensitive and specific, unless there is a concomitant haemothorax (especially left sided). The patient presenting in shock with a precordial wound warrants immediate operation. The anterior position of the heart places it at risk with a penetrating injury. In decreasing frequency, the cardiac chambers involved are 1. right ventricle, 2. left ventricle, 3. right atrium and 4. left atrium.

The chest is opened through a left anterolateral incision, with or without extension as a clamshell. It is the author's preference to immediately proceed with a clamshell if the patient is in shock or if there is a high suspicion for a cardiac injury. Compared to the anterolateral incision, the clamshell affords superior cardiac exposure, especially of the SVC, IVC and right atrium. It also allows the heart to be more easily delivered out of the pericardium and with less risk of injuring either phrenic nerve.

Once a myocardial injury is encountered, there are several techniques to obtain temporary bleeding control including digital pressure, myocardial closure with skin staples and placing a Foley catheter through the cardiac injury, followed by balloon inflation to occlude the hole. *While all of these techniques have their proponents the author's choice is direct, gentle digital pressure.* Staples may make the definitive repair more challenging and, if the Foley is placed under tension, it may pull out of the heart creating an even larger wound to repair. Once the injury is identified and temporary control obtained, plans for definitive repair are formulated. This also affords time for the anaesthesia team to 'catch up' with blood and blood product loss. In general, lower pressure structures – right atrium and ventricle – are easier to repair. The left atrium, although a relatively low-pressure chamber, is challenging to repair owing to its more posterior position within the chest. While both the IVC and SVC are low pressure, high flow structures, the intrathoracic IVC is quite short which presents a technical challenge to control and repair.

Right atrial and SVC injuries may be immediately controlled using a curved vascular clamp (**Figure 4.8**) and the injury closed with a running 4–0 or 5–0 polypropylene. If a more secure closure is necessary, then a two-layer closure is used: a deeper horizontal mattress suture and superficial running suture (author's preferred technique). The left atrium's posterior location can, as mentioned, present a challenge. A small, curved vascular clamp is very useful in maintaining control. The heart may need to be gently rotated to facilitate its repair. If doing this, warn the anaesthetic team, as manipulating the heart, especially with rotation, may cause severe haemodynamic compromise, particularly in the acidotic patient in severe shock. Care must be exercised during this manoeuvre and close communication with the anaesthesia team is essential.

The right ventricular pressure is about one quarter that of systemic, which facilitates the repair but its myocardium is thinner compared with the left ventricle, making it prone to tearing (suture may 'cheese-wire' through) if not carefully sutured. The left ventricle is under systemic pressure and has a thicker myocardium. Although there is much written about using pledgets to bolster the repair, there are no hard and fast rules. Pledgets will distribute the suture's tension more uniformly, which may be beneficial with a thinner or more friable myocardium. Attention to detail is paramount when repairing a ventricular wound.

The author's preference is interrupted, double armed 3–0 polypropylene, with pledgets as indicated. The choice of the needle is critical; a longer, more curved needle is ideal. *It is essential that the needle engages the ventricular wall at right angles, suture placement is timed*

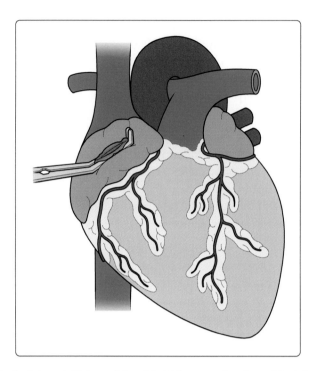

Figure 4.8 Control of a right atrial injury with a side-biting vascular clamp. The injury, once controlled, may then be over-run or under-run with 4–0 polypropylene (non-absorbable) suture.

to the ventricular contraction and the bite follows the curve of the needle. Keeping the systolic blood pressure less than 90 mmHg will aid suture placement. This is generally not a problem in the patient in shock but may require management in the resuscitated patient. Again, close cooperation and communication with the anaesthesia team is essential. Placing all the sutures prior to tying is also a useful technique. An intra-operative photograph of a left ventricular stab wound is demonstrated in **Figure 4.9**. A median sternotomy was performed and a pericardial sling constructed. A 1 cm laceration is seen just to the left of the left anterior descending (LAD) coronary artery. The repair is demonstrated in **Figure 4.10**.

Injuries adjacent to a coronary artery present a particular challenge. Small, distal coronary arterial branches can be ligated with minimal morbidity. However, ligation of a large, proximal coronary artery may prove fatal (massive myocardial infarction). Precise suture placement deep to the vessel will avoid narrowing or occluding the coronary vessel (**Figure 4.11**).

Injuries involving the posterior wall can also be problematic, since the heart needs to be rotated to visualise the posterior surface. During this manoeuvre there is frequently a precipitous drop in blood pressure and ventricular fibrillation is not uncommon. For any cardiac operation always have internal defibrillation paddles in the field. The approach to these injuries needs to be well-thought-out with a precise, deliberative repair. Once the posterior injury is rapidly identified the heart is returned to its normal position. The sutures should be ready-loaded on needle holders and placed through pledgets, if they are to be used. The heart is then manipulated allowing visualization of the injury and, the suture rapidly, but precisely, placed. The heart is again returned to its normal position with

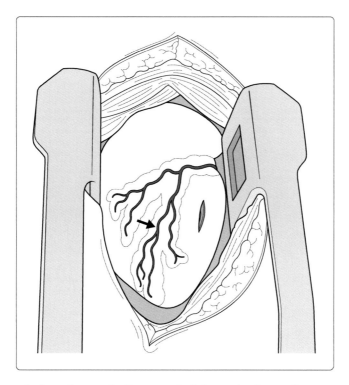

Figure 4.9 Left ventricular stab wound adjacent to the left anterior descending coronary artery (arrow).

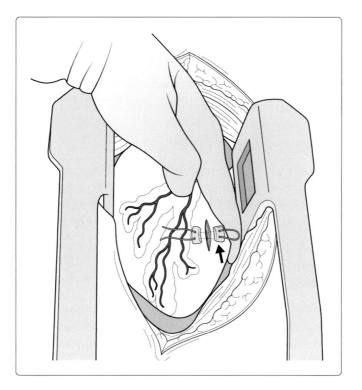

Figure 4.10 Repair of the left ventricular stab wound in **Figure 4.9** using pledgets (arrow).

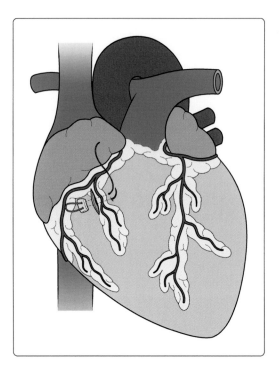

Figure 4.11 Ventricular injury in proximity to a coronary artery. The sutures are carefully placed deep to the vessel avoiding stenosis or occlusion.

resolution of profound hypotension. This process is repeated until all the sutures are in place and then repeated when tying. If an intra-cardiac injury (atrial septal defect, ventricular septal defect) is diagnosed (e.g. intraoperative trans-oesophageal echocardiography), repair is deferred. There is almost never a need for cardiopulmonary bypass when managing traumatic cardiac injuries. *The management of penetrating cardiac injuries demands rapid assessment, optimal exposure, a precise repair and close coordination with anaesthesia.*

Hilar injuries

Hilar injuries are typically severe , often requiring a formal anatomic pulmonary resection, and are associated with significant mortality and morbidity. The major concern with a hilar injury is life-threatening, freely exsanguinating haemorrhage, and less commonly air embolism. In either case, *hilar control* is essential. There are two common methods to rapidly control the hilum:

1. Pulmonary hilar twist
2. Direct manual control

Option number 2 is the authors preferred method of hilar vascular control. With the pulmonary hilar twist, the inferior pulmonary ligament is incised to allow mobilisation of the lung and the lobes rotated clockwise resulting in instant hilar in-flow control (**Figure 4.12**). For direct manual control, rapid blunt dissection enables the operator to control the hilum between the thumb and forefinger, and then place a vascular clamp for definitive control (**Figure 4.13**).

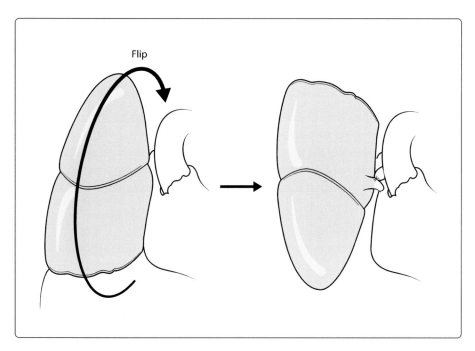

Figure 4.12 Pulmonary hilar twist. The lung is rotated clockwise occluding the hilar vessels. The acute increase in pulmonary vascular resistance and decrease pre-load may result in cardiovascular collapse.

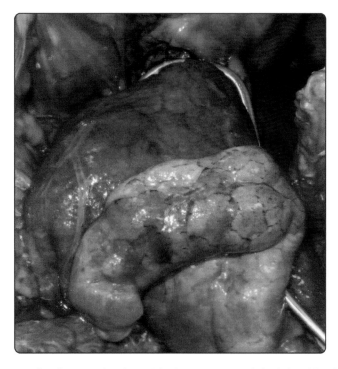

Figure 4.13 Hilar control with a vascular clamp. The lung is retracted, the hilum bluntly dissected and a vascular clamp applied. Haemodynamic compromise may occur.

With either technique, there may be sudden and dramatic haemodynamic changes as a result of loss of preload and rapid increase in pulmonary vascular resistance (50% of the pulmonary vascular space is acutely removed). Once haemorrhage has been controlled a detailed evaluation of the injury may be performed. Occasionally a hilar injury can be primarily repaired, but more typically an anatomic resection, lobectomy or pneumonectomy is necessary.

When performing a lobectomy or pneumonectomy it is preferable to isolate the pulmonary artery, pulmonary vein and bronchus separately. They can be individually divided using surgical staplers. Reinforcing the bronchial stump with a vascularised muscle pedicle (e.g. intercostal or diaphragm) will decrease the risk of a bronchial stump suture line dehiscence (bronchopleural fistula), which is associated with significant morbidity and mortality.

Pulmonary injuries

There are several techniques to manage pulmonary parenchymal injuries, and choosing the appropriate one depends on the severity of injury (typically depth of injury) and the patient's physiologic state. In the presence of profound shock, severe metabolic acidosis, coagulopathy and hypothermia, a damage control strategy is the optimal approach. Lung parenchymal trauma ranges from minimal (treated with suture repair) to severe (requiring a pneumonectomy). Simple, superficial pulmonary lacerations can be closed by pneumonorraphy (**Figure 4.14**). Through and through pulmonary injuries are managed by *tractotomy*. This is a simple, well-described, rapid method to control deeper lung lacerations not involving the hilum. A stapler is placed through the injury tract and fired (**Figure 4.15**). Once the tract is opened, air leaks from small airways and bleeding vessels are controlled with suture ligation. This is an excellent damage control technique. A non-anatomic wedge resection is another rapid method to address more extensive parenchymal injuries and is particularly suited to peripheral lung injuries. The lung is grasped with a lung clamp and a stapler fired to excise the injured lung. For a larger, non-anatomic resection, multiple reloads are typically necessary (**Figure 4.16**). The staple line is inspected for bleeding or

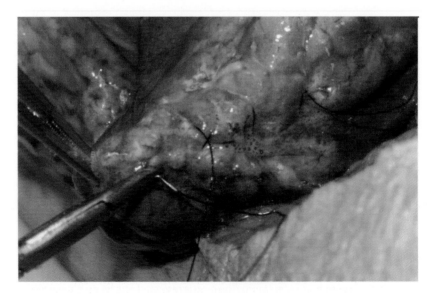

Figure 4.14 Pneumonorrhaphy with a running suture for a superficial lung laceration.

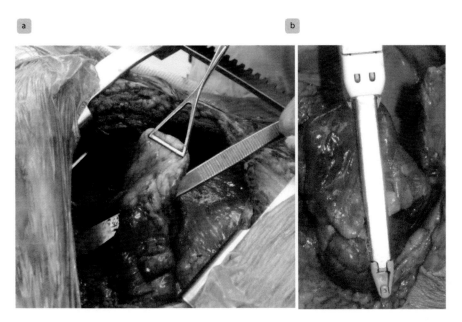

Figure 4.15 (a). A through and through lung injury is shown (the forceps has been placed through the lung defect for the purposes of demonstration); (b). A tractotomy is performed with a stapler. The GIA stapling device is then placed through the lung tubular defect and 'fired', thereby opening up the tract (tractotomy) whilst simultaneously sealing the cut edges of the lung. Any individual bleeding vessels may then be identified and ligated and the lung edges oversewed as necessary. The process may be repeated for deeper lung tracts.

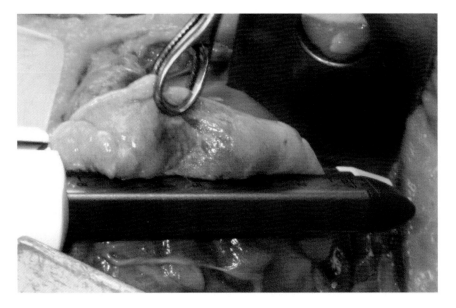

Figure 4.16 A stapled wedge resection. The GIA stapling device is placed across the lung, thereby isolating the injured segment and then 'fired' to remove the injured segment. The cut edge of lung may be oversewn (if required) for improved haemostasis. Multiple loads can be used if a more extensive non- anatomic resection is required.

gross air leak, which is then controlled by over-sewing the staple line. This technique is not appropriate if there is hilar involvement. In these instances, an anatomic resection, either lobectomy or pneumonectomy, is necessary.

If an anatomic resection is performed it is crucial to understand the pulmonary arterial and venous anatomy. A detailed description of all of these procedures is beyond the scope of this chapter, but the operative principles are careful dissection of the pulmonary arterial branches to the injured lobe with double-ligation before dividing them (or ligation with suture ligation (author's preference)), and individually dividing the pulmonary vein and bronchus with a stapler. The steps are the same for a pneumonectomy, however, the vessels and bronchus can be individually divided using a stapler. Muscle coverage of the bronchial stump is advised.

Posterior mediastinal injuries

The posterior structures at risk are

- Descending thoracic aorta
- Oesophagus
- Tracheobronchial tree

The descending thoracic aorta is approached through a left anterolateral or clamshell thoracotomy, however, the operative approach to the airway and oesophagus depends on the location of the injury. An anterolateral or clamshell approach provides adequate exposure for thoracic exploration in general, but is more limited for tracheobronchial tree and oesophageal exposure. Once an aero-digestive injury is diagnosed and its location determined, a postero-lateral thoracotomy is the preferred surgical approach.

Aortic injury

As discussed earlier, thoracic aortic exposure is enhanced by incising the inferior pulmonary ligament, retracting the lung anteriorly and widely opening the mediastinal pleura overlying the aorta. This exposes the thoracic aorta from the origin of the left subclavian artery down to the diaphragm. Haemorrhage is initially controlled with gentle digital pressure or by applying a partial occluding vascular clamp. Once temporary control is obtained, definitive repair can be accomplished using interrupted 3–0 or 4–0 polypropylene sutures. Even though the vessel has a relatively large lumen it is important not to stenose it during repair. More extensive injuries or those where a tension-free repair cannot be achieved, may require an interposition graft (but these injuries are more often fatal).

Tracheobronchial injury

Management of tracheobronchial injuries greatly depends on the site of injury. Flexible bronchoscopy is the diagnostic modality of choice and should be performed by the operative surgeon to precisely define the location of the injury. Proximal intra-thoracic airway injuries can be repaired through a collar incision, but injuries to the distal trachea, including the carina, the right bronchus and proximal left bronchus are repaired through a right postero-lateral thoracotomy. Conversely, distal left bronchial injuries are explored through a left postero-lateral thoracotomy. Tracheo-oesophageal injuries are one of the exceptions to a clamshell thoracotomy for exposure. This is the incision of choice for a surgical exploration but not well suited for posterior structures. The postero-lateral exposure is ideal for a definitive repair as opposed to the initial exploration for haemorrhage control.

Single lung ventilation with a double lumen endotracheal tube will greatly facilitate exposure in those patients who are being operated upon for trachea-oesophageal injuries, but has no role in patients who are in haemorrhagic shock or *in extremis*. The patient is positioned in the lateral decubitus position with an axillary roll in place. A standard curvilinear thoracotomy incision is made starting 2–3 finger breadths below the nipple, passing 2 finger breadths below the scapular tip and ending midway between the scapula and spine (**Figure 4.17**). The serratus anterior and latissimus dorsi muscles are divided with electrocautery (a muscle sparing approach can also be used). The ribs are counted and the pleural space entered in the 5th intercostal space. Since most tracheobronchial injuries are exposed from the right side, that approach will be discussed. The azygos vein is isolated, doubly ligated and divided. Then the mediastinal pleura is widely incised and can be tacked back to provide better exposure to the tracheobronchial tree (**Figure 4.18**). A nasogastric tube will facilitate defining the plane between the oesophagus and trachea. Care must be taken when mobilising the trachea as its blood supply is segmental. The trachea is debrided back to healthy tissue and repaired with interrupted absorbable sutures. Extreme care must be exercised to avoid puncturing the endotracheal tube balloon or catching the endotracheal tube with a suture. Early post-operative extubation is the goal.

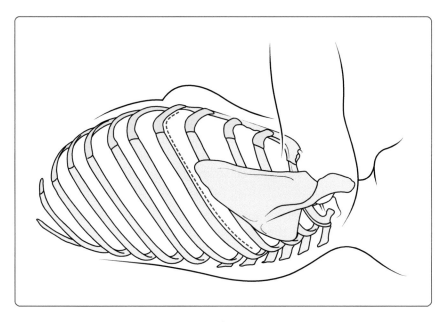

Figure 4.17 A postero-lateral thoracotomy. This is useful incision to repair tracheobronchial and oesophageal injuries but is not the incision of choice for initial emergency thoracic exploration. The incision starts 2–3 cm below the nipple and is carried in a curvilinear fashion following the line of the rib space, passing 2 finger breaths below the tip of the scapula and ending approximately half way between the scapula and the spine.

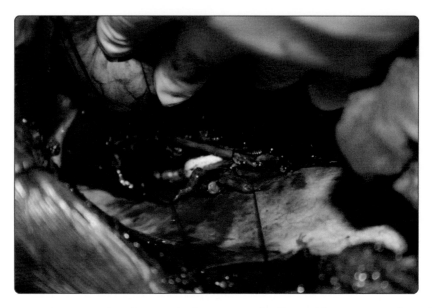

Figure 4.18 Intra-operative photograph of a severe tracheal injury. The exposure is through a right thoracotomy, the mediastinal pleura is retracted by tacking sutures and the endotracheal tube is plainly visible through the tracheal defect.

Oesophageal injury

A delayed diagnosis and/or management of an intra-thoracic oesophageal injury is associated with an extremely high mortality, secondary to mediastinitis and sepsis. Mediastinal air on chest radiograph or CT scan warrants further investigation. Given the proximity of the trachea and oesophagus both should be separately evaluated. Oesophageal injuries are diagnosed utilising both oesophagoscopy and an oesophagram. By combining both of these modalities, the accuracy in diagnosing an oesophageal injury approaches 100%. As with bronchoscopy, the operating surgeon should perform the endoscopy in order to precisely localise the injury. All but the most distal intra-thoracic oesophageal injuries (those near the oesophago-gastric junction) are approached through a right postero-lateral thoracotomy. The technical details for exploring the mediastinum are identical to those for a tracheobronchial injury. Oesophageal blood supply is sub-mucosal so the oesophagus can be widely mobilised. Its lack of a serosal layer demands a precise repair to avoid a post-operative leak.

Following debridement of non-viable tissue a two-layer closure is performed. Attention to detail is essential. The mucosa must be precisely re-approximated, the muscular layer sutures placed at a slightly oblique angle and all the knots tied on the outside. Corner stay sutures in addition to performing the repair over a nasogastric (NG) tube may be helpful adjuncts. **Figure 4.19** demonstrates a right postero-lateral approach to an intra-thoracic oesophageal injury, with the NG tube clearly visible. Wide drainage, distal feeding access, NPO and antibiotics are essential. The drains remain *in situ* until an oesophagram is performed, generally between the 7th and 14th post-operative day. If there is no leak the patient can eat and the drains are removed if there is no increased output.

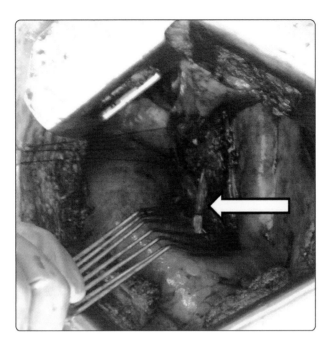

Figure 4.19 Intra-thoracic oesophageal injury. Exposure is through a right postero-lateral thoracotomy, tacking sutures retract the mediastinal pleura and the lung is retracted. The NG tube (arrow) is seen outside the oesophageal lumen.

Combined tracheobronchial injuries

The proximity of the trachea, oesophagus and great vessels make combined injuries likely. The strategy for dealing with this situation is to manage each injury as if it were in isolation. The crucial difference is to position a vascularised muscle buttress between the suture lines. This will nearly eliminate fistula formation between the adjacent suture lines, which could be a fatal complication.

Median sternotomy and control of arch vessels

Injury to the great vessels and the aortic arch can be particularly formidable. These injuries result in rapid, massive haemorrhage, and obtaining adequate exposure and control is challenging. There are two common surgical exposures to the arch and great vessels:

1. Median sternotomy
2. Clamshell thoracotomy

Each has advantages and disadvantages. Clamshell thoracotomy has already been discussed. If the incision is properly placed it affords adequate exposure of the superior mediastinum (**Figure 4.6**), however, if placed too inferiorly (a common problem) exposure will be less optimal. Median sternotomy provides excellent exposure of the heart and great vessels (**Figure 4.20**). It is also versatile and can be extended in to the neck, periclavicular region (supraclavicular) or into the abdomen as a laparotomy (**Figure 4.21**) as required. The major disadvantages are the surgeon's experience and the need for specialised

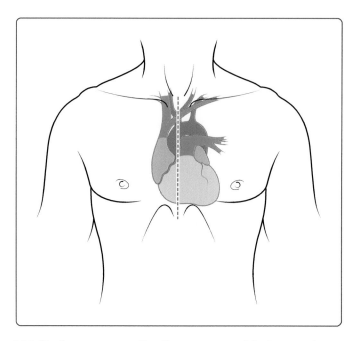

Figure 4.20 Median sternotomy. Excellent exposure of the heart and great vessels is obtained with this exposure. The incision is centered on the sternum and carried from the sternal notch to 1–2 cm below the xiphoid.

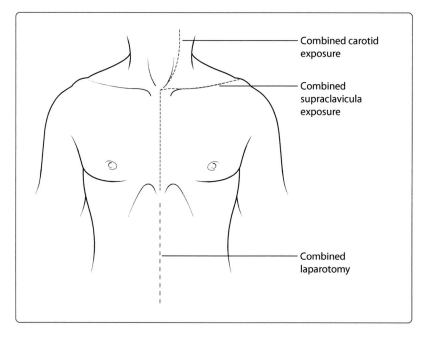

Combined carotid exposure

Combined supraclavicula exposure

Combined laparotomy

Figure 4.21 The median sternotomy is quite versatile and can be extended as depicted. It can also be continued as a laparotomy.

equipment (e.g. sternal saw). A skin incision extends from the sternal notch to 1–2 cm inferior to the xiphoid and using electrocautery the incision is deepened down to sternum. Blunt dissection at the sternal notch and the xiphoid will open a plane posterior to the sternum. Staying in the midline, the periosteum is scored and the sternum divided. Localising the midline is facilitated by palpating the lateral sternal borders. Incisions off the midline can be closed using a variety of techniques and it is always better to have a live patient who needs chest wall reconstruction than not.

Once exposure is obtained the vessels are explored. The gatekeeper to this region is the *left innominate vein*, which crosses *anterior* to the aortic arch and its branches. Once mobilised (or ligated), the arch vessels can be individually isolated and controlled. With the exception of the SVC and IVC, the great veins can be ligated. It is important to ensure that veins to be ligated do not have a central line! Arterial injuries may be initially controlled with gentle digital pressure until vascular clamps are applied. In the damage control situation, vascular shunts can be used and definitive reconstruction delayed until haemodynamic and physiologic stability is restored. Depending on the extent of the arterial injury, primary repair or interposition grafting is utilised.

There are a few key anatomic points:

- It is important to appreciate the location of the recurrent laryngeal nerves; the right encircles the proximal right subclavian artery and the left passes around the aortic arch between the left carotid and subclavian arteries
- There is also variation in the origin of the arch vessels; the most frequent variant is a common origin of the innominate and left common carotid arteries (bovine arch), but other arch anatomic anomalies also exist

Closure and drainage

The first decision is whether the thoracic cavity should be closed. If in damage control mode (profound shock, severe metabolic acidosis, coagulopathy and hypothermia), the chest may be packed open (**Figures 4.22 and 4.23**). Concerns that packing the pleural space will result in cardiac tamponade or compromised pulmonary function are unfounded. The technique is straightforward: pleural and mediastinal drains are placed, the pleural surfaces are packed with laparotomy pads and a modified vacuum dressing is applied. Posteriorly positioned, large bore (38 or 40 Fr) chest drains are essential. A smaller mediastinal drain (24 or 28 Fr), either straight or angled, is paced in the mediastinum. The author's approach is to place an angled mediastinal tube in the pericardium. Coagulopathic bleeding from the raw pleural surfaces are controlled with the laparotomy pads; avoid tightly packing against the mediastinum. A sterile 10 × 10 Steri-Drape (3M) is fenestrated and placed over the chest and mediastinal contents, including the lung and heart. Moist towels are placed over the Steri-Drape, two NG tubes are positioned on the towels and a large Ioban (3M) adhesive drape secures the dressing. A vacuum seal is achieved by applying suction to the NG tubes.

Following correction of the metabolic derangements (restoration of normal pH, clotting factors and temperature), the chest may be formally closed. This is typically performed

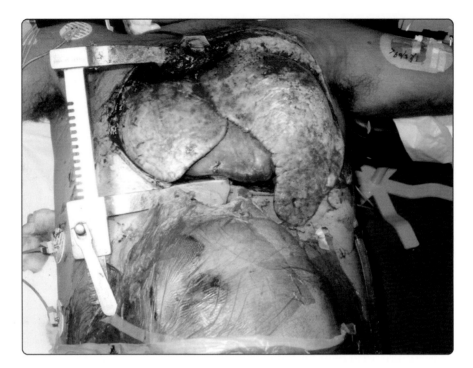

Figure 4.22 Damage control thoracic surgery. This patient sustained severe blunt trauma requiring a damage control laparotomy (modified closure is seen) and damage control clamshell.

on the second or third day following damage control. Generally, these patients are significantly volume overloaded and, once physiologically replete, diuresis is begun, which facilitates chest closure. On return to the operating room, the modified vacuum dressing and packs are carefully removed, and the pleural spaces irrigated removing fibrin deposits or retained haemothorax. Routine closure of the bony thorax is performed. The chest wall musculature may require debridement prior to closure and the skin is generally left open.

Anterolateral thoracotomy

If the patient is stable enough for chest closure, it is accomplished as it would for an elective procedure. The pleural space is irrigated after haemostasis has been achieved. Generally, two pleural tubes are placed, anterior and posterior with the tips near the apex. If there is concern for fluid accumulating inferiorly, an angled tube is positioned in the costophrenic angle. They are connected to individual collecting systems and placed on suction. The skeletal thorax is closed with interrupted, large (0 or #1) absorbable or non-absorbable sutures. Tension can be taken off the chest wall by pulling the sutures together prior to tying or by using a Bailey rib approximator. The muscle groups are closed in layers with running absorbable sutures and the skin closed with staples or sutures. Obtaining a portable chest radiograph prior to leaving the operating room is also preferable.

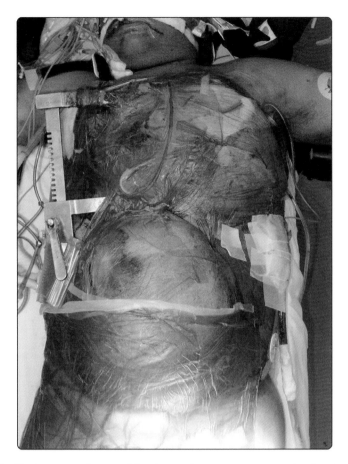

Figure 4.23 Modified vacuum closure of the thorax. Attempts to remove the chest retractor prior to modified closure resulted in profound hypotension, therefore, it was incorporated in the modified closure. Definitive chest closure was performed 3 days after the index operation. Following a prolonged hospitalisation the patient made a full recovery.

Clamshell

Clamshell closure is similar to closing an anterolateral thoracotomy with a few important differences. The sternum, which was divided horizontally, is closed with stainless steel wire, as a simple closure or figure of eight. Remember to ensure that the bilateral internal thoracic (mammary) arteries are ligated (proximally and distally). These vessels may not be bleeding briskly in the hypotensive patient and may be overlooked. Finally, the chest wall musculature becomes attenuated toward the midline and, occasionally, local advancement of the pectoralis is necessary to permit a tension-free closure.

Midline sternotomy

Sternotomy closure is accomplished as it would be or an elective operation. After obtaining haemostasis, small bore mediastinal drains are positioned, an angled tube placed over the diaphragm into the pericardium and a straight tube placed anteriorly. Typically, the pericardium is left open and the sternum closed with interrupted, figure of eight wire, taking care not to incorporate the anterior chest drain.

There is a difference of opinion about the utility of a pleural tube following an elective pneumonectomy: some surgeons place it while others prefer not to. Following a traumatic pneumonectomy, a pleural tube is useful, as there may be ongoing coagulopathic bleeding. *However, it is imperative that the pleural tube is placed on water seal and not suction.* Applying suction to the chest tube in this circumstance, which is in an empty hemithorax, may lead to mediastinal shift, which if severe results in profound hypotension and possible cardiovascular collapse (i.e. tension pneumothorax).

Chest tubes are left on suction until the air leak has resolved, then placed to water seal. Chest tubes are removed when the drainage is between 100 and 200 mL per day and mediastinal tubes when less than 50 mL/day.

Additional reading

Asensio JA, Berne JD, Demetriades D et al. One hundred give penetrating cardiac injuries: A 2-year prospective evaluation. *J Trauma* 1998;44:1073–1082.

Asensio JA, Chahwan S, Forno W et al. Penetrating esophageal injuries: Multicenter study of the American Association for the Surgery of Trauma. *J Trauma* 2001;50(2):289–296.

Asensio JA, Garcia-Nunez LM, Petrone P. Trauma to the heart. In Feliciano DV, Mattox KL, Moore EE, eds. *Trauma*. 6th ed. New York, NY: McGraw-Hill Medical, 2008;569–586.

Asensio JA, Murray J, Demetriades D et al. Penetrating cardiac injuries: A prospective study of variables predicting outcomes. *J Am Coll Surg* 1998;186:24–34.

Cassada DC, Munyikwa MP, Moniz MP, Dieter RA, Schuchmann GF, Enderson BL. Acute injuries of the trachea and major bronchi: Importance of early diagnosis. *Ann Thorac Surg* 2000;69:1563–1567.

Cothren C, Moore EE, Biffl WL, Franciose RJ, Offner PJ, Burch JM. Lung-sparing techniques are associated with improved outcome compared with anatomic resection for severe lung injuries. *J Trauma* 2002;53:483–487.

DuBose J, O'Connor JV, Scalea TM. Lung, trachea and esophagus. In Feliciano DV, Mattox KL, Moore EE, eds. *Trauma*. 7th ed. New York: McGraw Hill, 2013;468–484.

Fulton JO, de Groot KM, Buckels NJ, von Oppell UO. Penetrating injuries involving the intrathoracic great vessels. *S Afr J Surg* 1997;35:82–86.

Goins WA, Ford DH. The lethality of penetrating cardiac wounds. *Am Surg* 1996;62(12):987–993.

Hajarizadeh H, Rohrer MJ, Cutler BS. Surgical exposure of the left subclavian artery by median sternotomy and left supraclavicular extension. *J Trauma* 1996;41:136–139.

Huh J, Wall MW Jr, Estrera AL, Soltero ER, Mattox KL. Surgical management of traumatic pulmonary injury. *Am J Surg* 2003;186:620–624.

Karmy-Jones R, Jurkovich GJ, Nathens AB et al. Timing of urgent thoracotomy for hemorrhage after trauma. *Arch Surg* 2001;36:513–8.

Karmy-Jones R, Jurkovich GJ, Shatz DV et al. Management of traumatic lung injury: A western trauma association multicenter review. *J Trauma* 2001;51:1049–1053.

Mandal KS, Sanusi M. Penetrating chest wounds: 24 years experience. *World J Surg* 2001;25:1145–1149.

Martin MJ, McDonald JM, Mullenix PS, Steele SR, Demetriades D. Operative management and outcomes of traumatic lung resection. *J Am Coll Surg* 2006;203:336–344.

Meredith JW, Hoth JJ. Thoracic trauma: When and how to intervene. *Surg Clin North Am* 2007;87:95–118.

O'Connor JV, DuBose JJ, Scalea TM. Damage control thoracic surgery: Management and outcomes. *J Trauma Acute Care Surg* 2014;77(5):660–665.

O'Connor JV, Scalea TM. Penetrating thoracic great vessel injury: Impact of admission hemodynamics and preoperative imaging. *J Trauma* 2010;68(4):834–837.

Rhee PM, Acosta J, Bridgeman A, Wang D, Jordan M, Rich N. Survival after emergency department thoracotomy: Review of published data from the past 25 ears. *J Am Coll Surg* 2000;190:288–298.

Rossbach MM, Johnson SB, Gomez MA, Sako EY, Miller OL, Calhoon JH. Management of major tracheobronchial injuries: A 28-year experience. *Ann Thorac Surg* 1998;65:182–186.

Rotondo MF, Schwab CW, McGonigal MD et al. 'Damage control': An approach for improved survival in exsanguinating penetrating abdominal injury. *J Trauma* 1993;35(3):375–382.

Smakman N, Nicol AJ, Walther G, Brooks A, Navsaria PH, Zellweger R. Factors affecting outcome in penetrating oesophageal trauma. *Br J Surg* 2004;91(11):1513–1519.

Tominaga GT, Waxman K, Scannell G, Annas C, Ott RA, Gazzaniga AB. Emergency thoracotomy with lung resection following trauma. *Am Surg* 1993;59(12):834–837.

Tyburski JG, Astra L, Wilson RF, Dente C, Staffes C. Factors affecting prognosis with penetrating wounds of the heart. *J Trauma* 2000;48:587–590; discussion 590–591.

Von Oppell UO, Bautz P, De Groot M. Penetrating thoracic injuries: What we have learnt. *Thorac Cardiovasc Surg* 2000;48:55–61.

5 Vascular Trauma

Morgan McMonagle

Mechanism of vascular injury

Vascular injuries may be *blunt*, *penetrating* (high versus low energy) or *iatrogenic*. For both blunt and penetrating injuries, the injuring force is directed from the external environment (i.e. out to in), passing through the surrounding tissues, with a higher likelihood of additional associated injury including additional bleeding and haematoma formation within the tissues (in addition to the vascular injury itself). Injured vessels (typically large named vessels) will have perivascular, surrounding haematoma (on imaging) or traumatic streaking in the adventitial plane (even if small). An iatrogenic injury however, typically results from injury during an endovascular procedure (or other vessel instrumentation) and may not have the same pattern of surrounding haematoma and inflammation (unless the vessel wall itself is fully traversed by the instrument) and may be confined to a small intimal tear or luminal irregularity only.

Penetrating injury may cause partial or complete laceration of the vessel (**Figure 5.1**). In the young patient, often a complete laceration will spasm closed, thereby slowing the rate of bleeding (especially when combined with hypotension). Partial lacerations on the other hand often remain widely patent, unable to 'spasm' closed with continuous, high flow bleeding.

Blunt injury may present as trauma and haemorrhage within the vessel wall only, with varying degrees of spasm, intimal tearing (flap), vessel wall haematoma and occlusion and thrombosis. Complete rupture of the vessel from blunt trauma is often associated with extensive tissue injury and free haemorrhage and other severe associated injuries (e.g. traumatic brain injury [TBI], chest, spine).

Epidemiology

Significant (i.e. requiring emergency surgery) vascular trauma only accounts for about 2%–3% of injuries overall, but represents the most challenging of conditions to manage, due to the risk of *rapid exsanguination* combined with difficulty gaining rapid *surgical access and control* of the vessel. Overall, vascular trauma is associated with a mortality >50% when a *non-compressible* body part is involved (e.g. abdomen, thorax, thoracic outlet), an overall stroke rate of 30%–50% with carotid artery injuries and a limb loss rate of 10% for peripheral vascular injury.

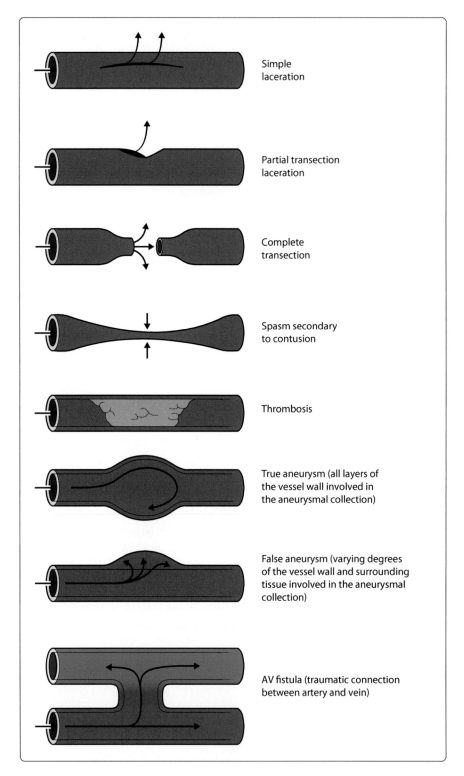

Figure 5.1 Variety of vascular injuries.

However, many vascular injuries (if they survive to reach hospital) are amenable to appropriate management (and repair) with restoration of normal haemodynamics and a successful outcome, even with simple manoeuvres performed by a non-specialist surgeon.

> The biggest risk after vascular trauma is massive haemorrhage

Massive haemorrhage quickly leads to a spiralling decline in physiology and metabolic status with a combination of *hypothermia, coagulopathy* and *acidosis* ('triad of death'). **Expedient haemorrhage control (even by the non-vascular specialist) will rapidly reverse (or avoid) this triad and is key to survival, limb salvage and a good neurological outcome.**

Anatomical challenges in vascular trauma

Consider the management of vascular injuries broadly as;

1. Compressible (upper and lower limbs)
2. Non-compressible (chest, abdominal and pelvic cavities)
3. Semi-compressible (neck)

Active bleeding in a compressible region may be temporised with a combination of simple external manoeuvres such as direct manual compression, tourniquet (TK) application and compression dressings in advance of operative (or occasionally interventional radiology [IR]) control. The hard signs (see later) of vascular injury apply to this group of injuries. Non-compressible cavity haemorrhage will require rapid decision making for operative control (perhaps augmented by IR input) and the hard signs of vascular injury do not apply. Semi-compressible bleeding occurs in the neck, and although external compression may be applied, care must be taken not to occlude the carotid arteries or the airway. Some of the hard signs apply here, but emergent rapid sequence intubation (RSI) and operative control is the preferable approach.

The junctional zones

A junctional zone describes *two or more juxtaposed body regions*. Structures, especially vascular, in one zone will typically traverse into the adjacent zone, whereby an injury on one area carries a high likelihood of an associated concomitant injury in this neighbouring zone (especially penetrating injury). In addition, the junctional zones also have challenging surgical anatomy that is difficult to 'access' rapidly for bleeding control. Thus, vascular injuries in a non-compressible junctional zone are associated with a high risk of exsanguination and surgical control often involves dual access to both juxtaposed zones simultaneously. The junctional zones are;

• Thoraco-cervical zone (root of the neck/thoracic outlet)
• Thoraco-abdominal zone (base of the rib cage)
• Pelvis–lower limb (groin)

Injuries at the root of the neck (or any vascular neck injury) may require proximal control from within the chest. Injuries to the thoraco-abdominal zone may involve both the thorax and abdomen, thereby challenging the surgeon as to the order of cavity (both non-compressible) exploration.

Proximal lower limb vascular (iliac) injuries (*inflow* to the lower limb) are non-compressible and challenging to safely dissect and control proximally (i.e. within the pelvis). TKs are typically ineffective here, as they cannot be placed high enough for adequate compression and in fact may aggravate bleeding if placed too distal to the injury. Proximal control is best achieved within the pelvis *via* extraperitoneal dissection (or transperitoneal if a laparotomy is already in progress). *If the physiology is subnormal or the patient is in extremis, then a rapid antero-lateral thoracotomy with cross-clamping of the descending thoracic aorta is the easiest, quickest and most effective way to gain vascular control of bleeding* (see Chapter 4).

Decision-making in vascular trauma

Decision-making in trauma (especially with active haemorrhage) is determined by *patient physiology*. Physiologically unwell patients (often colloquially referred to as 'unstable') mandate immediate surgical management. Patients who are physiologically within normal limits can be afforded time to undergo further investigations as indicated. Computed tomography (CT) scanning for the trauma patient is now a well-established investigation in Western healthcare, enabling the treating surgeon to identify life-threatening injuries early. However, it is important to appreciate that any patient presenting with hard signs of vascular injury (see next section) should undergo immediate surgical management (or occasionally endovascular management) without the need for further diagnostic workup (save for an on-table angiogram as indicated).

Hard versus soft signs of vascular injury

Hard signs of vascular injury are clinical signs that represent either arterial *bleeding* or arterial *ischaemia* (or both) and if present mandate further operative management without the need for diagnostic investigations (*Table 5.1*). They are an *absolute indication* of the presence of *significant* vascular injury, as they represent either *active arterial bleeding* or *absolute distal ischaemia*. Operative management is mandatory! The hard signs are;

- Loss of distal pulses (with or without other signs of distal ischaemia) → occluded vessel
- Pulsatile/expansile haematoma → arterial haemorrhage
- Palpable thrill or audible bruit → arterial haemorrhage (difficult to appreciate if very hypotensive)

Table 5.1 Hard versus soft signs of vascular injury

Hard signs (high sensitivity and specificity)	Soft signs (low sensitivity and specificity)
• Active arterial haemorrhage • Expanding/pulsatile haematoma • Bruit/thrill over haematoma • Loss of distal pulses	• History of bleeding • Injury in close proximity to a vessel • Non-pulsatile haematoma • Non-pulsatile bleeding • Neurological deficit • Unexplained hypotension • Diminished (but not absent) pulse

Soft signs are anything else that is not a hard sign, and they have a low sensitivity and specificity for significant arterial trauma. The soft signs are a mixed bag of clinical findings and may include; an injury or trajectory in close proximity to a vessel, history of bleeding on scene, non-pulsatile bleeding, non-pulsatile haematoma, nerve deficit and unexplained hypotension. In the absence of hard signs of vascular injury, significant arterial injury is unlikely, although minimal vascular injury may still be present (see next section).

It should also be remembered that the hard and soft signs are best applied to the extremities and obviously do not predict vascular injury in the chest or abdominal or pelvis (i.e. the non-compressible cavities). In addition, carotid injury may display classic hard signs, but detecting the loss of a pulse distal in the carotid is difficult and therefore a high index of suspicion is required for vascular injuries in any region where the hard signs do not apply.

Minimal vascular injury (MVI)

Minimal vascular injury (MVI) describes documented (typically on imaging) 'minor' vessel injury *without* hard signs (**Figure 5.2**). It is typically picked up incidentally during investigations (e.g. angiogram, Duplex) and injury is commonly confined to the intimal layer only. There are four recognised subtypes (*Table 5.2*):

- Focal segmental narrowing
- Intimal flap/irregularity
- Small pseudoaneurysm
- Arteriovenous (AV) fistula

The important characteristic of MVI is that there is *no active arterial bleeding* outside the vessel in addition to preservation of adequate antegrade flow and *no distal ischaemia* (i.e. no hard signs). The natural history of untreated MVI is well described in the literature and simple observation appears to be the management of choice, as the vast majority (>90%) will heal spontaneously. About 10% of cases will progress and develop symptoms which may require treatment, but which may be managed on an elective or semi-elective basis, with no documented increase in either mortality or morbidity. Of the four categories of MVIs, pseudoaneurysms are most likely to progress and become symptomatic compared to the others. Small pseudoaneurysms (<2 cm) picked up incidentally may be safely monitored, although 40%–50% greater than 2 cm will progress to symptoms requiring treatment. But even these may be safely observed for a time.

Early management of vascular injuries

All trauma patients are examined and managed *as per* the Advanced Trauma Life Support (ATLS®) guidelines of the American College of Surgeons. Maintain a high index of suspicion for vascular injuries due to the potential for rapid exsanguination, especially if a non-compressible cavity is involved and may be guided by the mechanism of injury (e.g. trans-abdominal gunshot wound, open-book pelvic fracture). In addition, any patient with hard signs of vascular injury mandates immediate surgical exploration. In short, any haemodynamically unwell, or those with hard signs, the standard ATLS approach must be abbreviated and postponed until after the life- (or limb) threatening injuries have been safely managed, as appropriate.

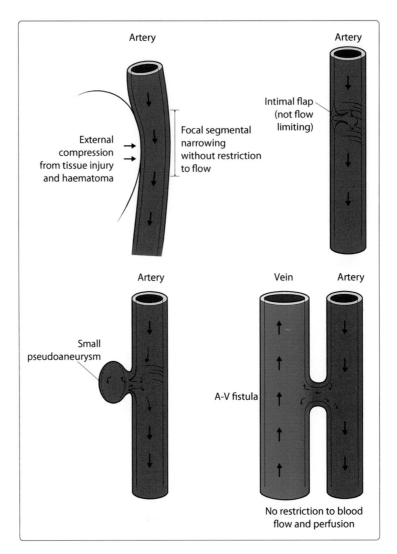

Figure 5.2 Minimal vascular injury.

Table 5.2 Minimal vascular injury

Type	Characteristics
1. Focal segmental narrowing	Smooth, regular narrowing with no constriction to flow. It may be caused by external compression, vessel wall haematoma or reactive spasm.
2. Intimal flap or irregularity	Small tear in intima protruding into lumen. The flap may be raised with either an antegrade or retrograde orientation, but there is no obstruction to luminal flow.
3. Pseudoaneurysm	Incomplete laceration of vessel with contained bleeding into a small volume of surrounding tissue, probably <2 cm.
4. AV fistula	Simultaneous lacerations in adjacent and juxtaposed artery and vein that actively communicate without passing through the capillary bed, probably <1.5 cm.

> Any patient presenting with hard signs of vascular injury mandates immediate operative intervention

Vascular injuries do not require large volume fluid resuscitation. It is better if actively bleeding patients are permitted to become relatively hypotensive ('permissive hypotension' or 'resuscitative hypotension') as a 'bridge' to definitive surgical haemostasis. *The actively bleeding poly-trauma patient only requires a survivable blood pressure (SBP 80–90 mm Hg) and not a normal blood pressure!* It is the 'time to haemostasis' that is the single most important determinant of survival in the actively bleeding patient. Hypotensive resuscitation minimises blood loss prior to surgical haemorrhage control.

> Time to haemostasis is the single biggest determinant for survival in the actively bleeding patient

Higher pressures, when artificially created with fluid and vasoconstrictors/inotropic agents, run the risk of dislodging the already vital but unstable thrombus at the site of bleeding (*'pop the clot' syndrome*), thereby encouraging further haemorrhage. In addition, fluids (crystalloid and colloids), will further aggravate a dilutional coagulopathy and contribute to hypothermia. If fluid resuscitation is used, use blood and blood products, administered through a warming device (level 1 fluid warmer).

> Actively bleeding patients require a 'survivable' blood pressure *en route* to the operating room and not a 'normal' blood pressure

The surgeon must also decide the order of injury priority when other 'competing' injuries coexist, especially in the presence of TBI at the time of going to the operating room. However, in general significant vascular injury incurs the highest priority.

Massive exsanguination

For the bleeding patient *in extremis* who is not yet in the operating room, the most rapid and immediate method of haemorrhage control is *via* a trauma bay thoracotomy (or clamshell thoracotomy) with cross-clamping of the descending thoracic aorta.

General approach to operative management

The operating room must be well equipped with both major vascular and general surgery instruments suitable for both chest and abdominal exploration. The operating room must be warm (30°C) to avoid and treat hypothermia, which itself is an independent predictor of mortality. The blood cell saver (if available) should be primed and ready for use and a level 1 fluid warmer used when administering blood. Cold blood or room-temperature fluids must be avoided in bleeding patients, as this will aggravate both coagulopathy and hypothermia (**Figure 5.3**).

Rapid infuser   Cell saver

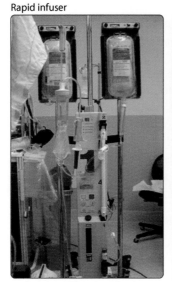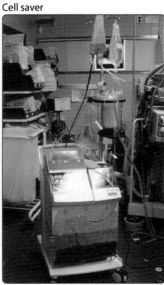

Figure 5.3 Rapid fluid infuser (which also warms fluids to body temperature) and cell saver (autotransfuser) used in surgery where there is a high risk of rapid exsanguination.

Individual staff members are assigned dedicated tasks by the lead trauma surgeon to which they are solely responsible (e.g. blood checking and administration, anaesthetic support, circulating for equipment). Close communication with anaesthetic staff is important, especially at critical times (e.g. simultaneous intubation and initiation of surgery). The patient is prepped from the base of the neck to the knees for access to all body cavities with both arms extended outwards for intravenous and arterial lines access ('crucifix' position; **Figure 5.4**).

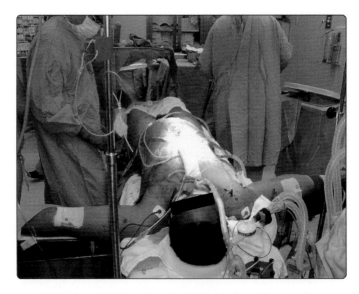

Figure 5.4 Patient in 'crucifix' position for full access to all body regions, especially chest–abdomen–pelvis.

Warming devices over the patient are cumbersome and unnecessary if the ambient temperature is maintained at 30°C, although a thermal warmer below the patient may be a useful addition.

If not already intubated, induction of anaesthesia in the bleeding patient is a co-ordinated effort between the anaesthetic staff and surgeon, using a reduced dose of induction agent (to avoid further worsening the hypotension) and the RSI should occur at the same time and in parallel with the 'first cut' of surgery. This is particularly true for major non-compressible cavity bleeding. The first incision is made as the intubating physician communicates that the endotracheal tube has passed through the vocal cords. This communication pattern is a continuous exercise and the surgeon should be kept up to date at regular intervals with regard to the patient's vital signs and other measurable parameters of the triad of death (pH, bicarbonate levels, base excess, coagulation profile and temperature), which may guide whether surgery should be abbreviated. In addition, the anaesthetist should be informed about injury findings and if / when adequate haemorrhage control has been achieved. In the physiologically unwell patient, direct and rapid opening of the bleeding cavity with sharp dissection is the preferred approach, as slower dissection with electrocautery only serves to delay gross haemorrhage control.

Surgical approach to vascular injuries

Dissection and control of vascular injuries

Typically, dissection and control of an injured vessel follows the following sequence:

1. Proximal vessel dissection and control first (through uninjured tissue).
2. Distal vessel dissection and control (through uninjured tissue).
3. 'Attack the injury': open the haematoma, expose vessel injury, then decide on best management (**Figure 5.5**).

Vessel handling

Utilise minimal handling to reduce further injury and thrombosis, and try to pick the vessel up by the adventitia only, using non-toothed vascular forceps. Once opened, never handle the vessel intima or pick it up with an instrument which will only cause an intimal tear and thrombosis.

Control of the vessel

A vascular 'loop' is carefully slung around the vessel (preferably a double loop) both above and below the injured segment (i.e. 'looping' or 'Pottsing' the vessel) (**Figure 5.6**). Once looped, this allows easy manipulation of the vessels without traumatising it in addition to allowing immediate control of bleeding by elevating the vascular loop tightly which in turn will 'snug-down' and compress the lumen of the vessel in an atraumatic fashion.

Large branches are controlled in this way, whilst smaller branches may be looped with a surgical tie (without actually tying a knot so as to preserve collateral supply) or with a temporarily placed ligaclip. Once looped, an appropriately sized vascular clamp is applied to the vessel for complete control of bleeding, thereby allowing the surgeon to confidently manage the injury without the fear of exsanguination upon opening the haematoma or injury.

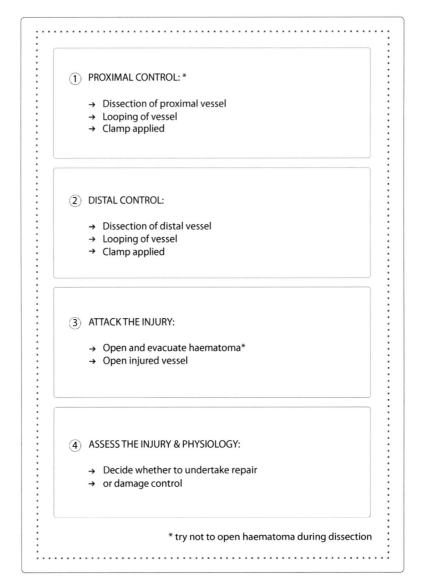

Figure 5.5 Approach to vascular injury.

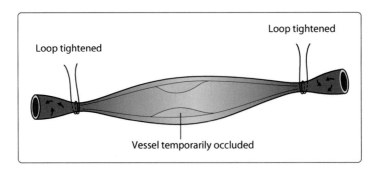

Figure 5.6 Tightening the loop.

Decision time

Once proximal and distal control are achieved, the injured tissue is opened, the haematoma evacuated and the vessel inspected. The surgeon must then decide on;

- Definitive repair
- Damage control

The decision is based on

1. Patient physiology (think 'deadly triad')
2. Injury burden (*predicted clinical course* of developing worsening physiology)
3. Concomitant ortho-vascular injuries
4. Your skill set!

Damage control for vascular trauma

- Ligation of vessel
- Primary amputation
- Shunting of the vessel

Acute ligation of a vessel is generally reserved for patients *in extremis* as shunt insertion is now the preferable option being both quick and effective.

Ligation of the vessel and primary amputation

Any vessel may be ligated acutely in the face of worsening haemodynamics and physiology, but the consequences of ligation may be catastrophic. *Table 5.3* describes the risk and complications of acute ligation. Remember, however, that the data shown pertains to acute arterial ligation in the non-shocked, non-traumatised patient, and therefore the risks of distal ischaemia and morbidity will be even higher with severe injury.

A primary amputation is rarely performed in modern trauma practice. If a patient is *in extremis* with a non-salvageable limb, a primary amputation takes much longer than

Table 5.3 Risk of distal ischaemia (or stroke rate in carotid artery ligation)

Vessel	Ischaemia risk (%)
Subclavian	15–20
Axillary	25–30
Brachial	30–40
Common carotid	10–15
Internal carotid	40–50
Common femoral	80
Superficial femoral	30–50
Popliteal	80

Note: In addition, an injured forearm vessel may be ligated if the other is intact. For vascular limb injuries below the knee, only one tibial vessel is required for adequate perfusion (but preferably not the peroneal artery). Ironically, the risk of lower limb loss rate is only 10%–15% if the CFA is ligated in intravenous drug use (IVDU) patients, due to the chronic ischaemia and collateral supply development.

acute ligation of bleeding vessels and leads to additional tissue destruction in the face of worsening physiology. In such a scenario, it is better to acutely ligate the vessel and await demarcation of the tissue over 24–48 hours (if the patient survives) and plan a return to surgery for delayed amputation at an appropriate level.

Shunting of the vessel

A shunt is any sterile, artificial tubing or conduit placed inside a vessel to permit continuous prograde perfusion. Although there are numerous commercially available shunts licenced for the carotid (as they are often used during a carotid endarterectomy) such as Pruitt-Inahara™, Javid™, Sundt™, Argyle™, any sterile tubing (typically plastic or sialastic for malleability) may be used such as a large bore nasogastric [NG] tube, Foley catheter, large angiocath, small chest drain. The following applies to safe shunt insertion:

- Choose an appropriate sized shunt/plastic tubing that will fit 'comfortably' inside the vessel. If too wide, it will not insert easily and will likely lift an intimal flap, causing acute thrombosis. If too small, it may leak or lead to increased resistance to flow with acute thrombosis.
- Cut the plastic tubing so that it fits comfortably. The shunt should typically have just enough 'redundancy' outside the vessel ends to allow some movement without the risk of slippage or kinking (especially if bony manipulation by orthopaedics is planned), but not too short (or it will slip out) or too long (which will add to flow resistance and thrombosis). A gentle external loop of the shunt is appropriate in the limb with dual vascular-orthopaedic injury (to allow manipulation and reduction of the fracture as the external fixator is applied). In a more protected cavity (e.g. abdomen, pelvis) where orthopaedic manipulation of bone is not necessary, then a shorter, straight shunt may be used.
- Ensure there is good 'inflow' from the vessel above. Briefly allow blood to flow from the proximal vessel (briefly open the vascular clamp). This will evacuate any thrombus proximally and prevent 'air locking'.
- Ensure good 'backflow' in the vessel below the injured segment. In addition, a balloon (e.g. Fogarty) catheter should be inserted distally and inflated whilst slowly withdrawing and any thrombus or debris removed. This should improve backflow from the distal vessel, seen as rapid back filling and retrograde blood flow from the distal vessel (typically non-pulsatile flow). Then copiously flush the distal vessel with heparinised saline to ensure good run-off.
- Bevel the ends of the shunt slightly to allow easier insertion. Take care not to lift an intimal flap during insertion. In addition, in young people, the intima may retract away from the vessel edge. Ensure it is visualised so that an intimal flap is not missed.
- The shunt is then tied in place proximally with a suture (preferably braided suture to prevent 'cheese-wiring' through the vessel wall) (**Figure 5.7**).
- Again, blood is briefly allowed to 'flush through' the shunt from proximal to release any debris (e.g. thrombus) and to prevent air locking.
- The distal end of the shunt is then inserted in the same manner into the distal portion of the vessel and tied *in situ* as before.
- Avoid systemic heparinisation in the polytrauma, coagulopathic patient, especially if a traumatic brain injury is present. However, the use of heparinised saline flushed locally into the injured vessel is safe.

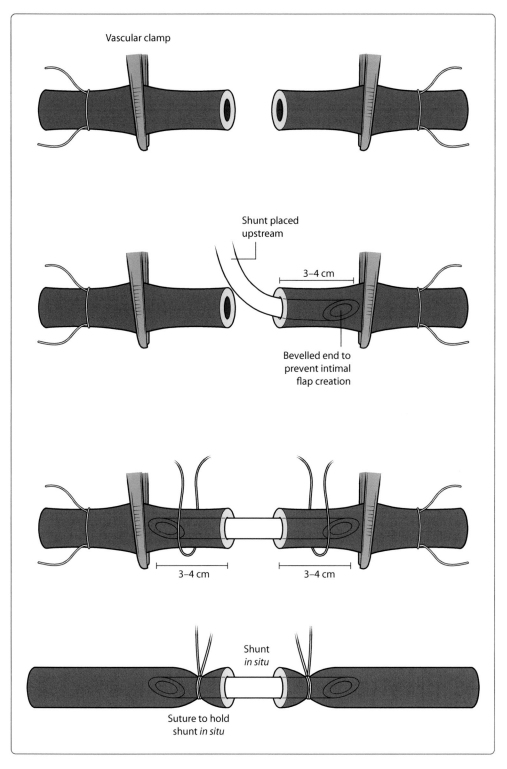

Figure 5.7 Vascular shunt insertion.

Shunt removal   Aim to remove the shunt as soon as possible to prevent acute thrombosis and distal ischaemia. Typically, this will be during damage control surgery (DCS) stage III after physiology has normalised, but it may need to be removed sooner if a shunt complication has occurred (e.g. occlusion) or after orthopaedic repair (if the shunt was inserted to facilitate this in the face of concomitant ortho-vascular injury, but normal physiology). Although shunts have been left *in situ* for prolonged periods, ideally aim to correct physiology and remove the shunt inside 6–12 hours. There is good evidence that shunts left longer than this are associated with an exponential rise in complications. Remember, when the shunt is removed and definitive repair planned, the segment of artery where the ligation tie was placed (which was previously normal uninjured vessel) also needs to be excised prior to repair as it has now been iatrogenically injured and crushed by the stay tie.

Is anti-coagulation necessary?   In the literature, shunts have been reportedly left *in situ* for 52 and 48 hours with and without anti-coagulation respectively. We would generally recommend against the use of systemic anticoagulation if a shunt is used during damage control surgery, as these patients are typically already coagulopathic from their injuries, especially in the first 24 hours. The important thing is to leave the distal limb exposed to assess regularly for worsening ischaemia and acute occlusion of the shunt and to take appropriate action (**Figure 5.8**).

Definitive vascular repair

Potential surgical repair techniques include:

- Patch grafting
- Direct end-to-end anastomosis
- Interposition grafting
- Vascular bypass
  - Autologous vein
    - Reversed vein
    - *In situ* vein
  - Synthetic
    - Dacron
    - ePTFE

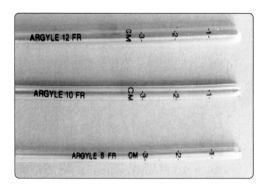

Figure 5.8 Selection of Argyle shunts for use in vascular surgery.

Figures **5.9** and **5.10** illustrate the various vascular techniques that may be employed, depending on the situation. However, in the setting of damage control, a definitive repair should not be undertaken, as further complex, additional bleeding and prolonged surgery will likely lead to a rapid demise in patient physiology. In addition, in the hypotensive coagulopathic patient, a definitive vascular repair is much more likely to fail, bleed or thrombose.

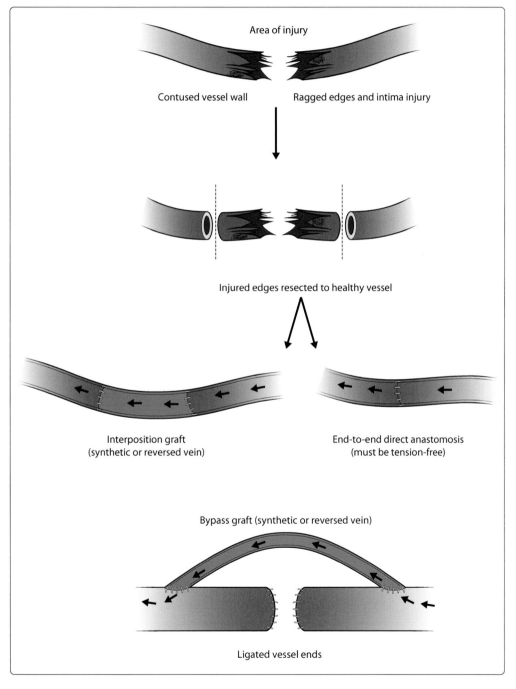

Figure 5.9 Arterial repair techniques (complete thickness injuries).

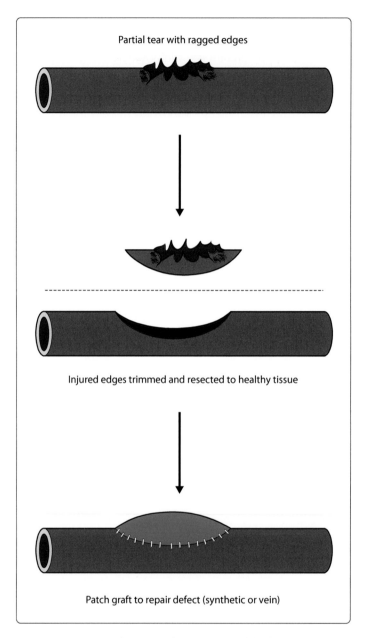

Partial tear with ragged edges

Injured edges trimmed and resected to healthy tissue

Patch graft to repair defect (synthetic or vein)

Figure 5.10 Arterial repair techniques (partial thickness injuries).

Whichever repair technique is used, there must be adequate inflow (above) and backflow/run-off (below). Vessels should also be intermittently 'flushed' with heparinised saline to remove debris and microthrombi from the circuit. Also ensure that the intima has not retracted into the vessel during repair (common in young patients) and that it is incorporated correctly into the anastomotic suture. A detailed description of vascular reconstruction and repair is beyond the scope of this book.

Performing the surgery

Emergency operative control follows the same pattern as elective surgery but performed in a more progressive and rapid fashion. As mentioned earlier, gain proximal vessel control first and loop it with a vascular sling so that it may be elevated by an assistant prior to clamping (**Figure 5.11**). If there is active haemorrhage at this stage, then a vascular clamp should be applied (**Figure 5.12**).

Then distal vessel dissection and control is performed, below the injury and the vessel double-looped. Once controlled and clamped, the injured tissue / haematoma is opened directly to expose the injured vessel. The normal dissection planes are often distorted by the combination of tissue destruction and expanding haematoma, but blunt manual dissection will guide the surgeons finger to the vessel as typically the haematoma has performed most of the dissection between planes already. Heparin should be avoided in the bleeding patient, as many of these patients are already coagulopathic. Major venous injuries may be approached in the same way as arterial and controlled, although direct dissection without proximal and distal control is also acceptable as venous bleeding (low pressure) may be readily controlled with direct pressure alone.

The injured artery is then inspected and the ends surgically trimmed, taking care not to cause additional trauma to the intimal layer (prone to re-coil into the vessel in young people which may create a dissection flap if not recognised). Small, single injuries on the vessel wall may be sutured directly or repaired with a vein patch if stenosis is a concern (**Figure 5.10**). However, more typically the vessel will require mobilisation and the injured portion resected (**Figure 5.9**). If a tension-free anastomosis between the trimmed ends is possible after mobilisation, then a direct anastomosis may be performed, but this is typically not possible. More often, grafting is required, either with an interposition graft or ligation of the vessel with bypass (**Figure 5.9**). Venous injuries may be ligated, especially if *in extremis*. However, we would advocate venous repair in the injured limb and inferior vena cava (IVC) where possible to reduce post-ligation side effects (see later).

The choice of material for grafting may be either an autologous vein (e.g. long saphenous vein) or synthetic. This will depend on the physiologic state of the patient and associated

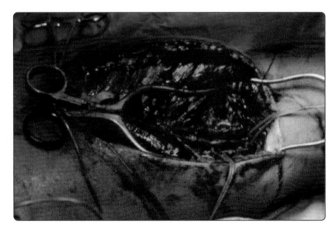

Figure 5.11 Dissection of left SFA with looping of vessel to control artery.

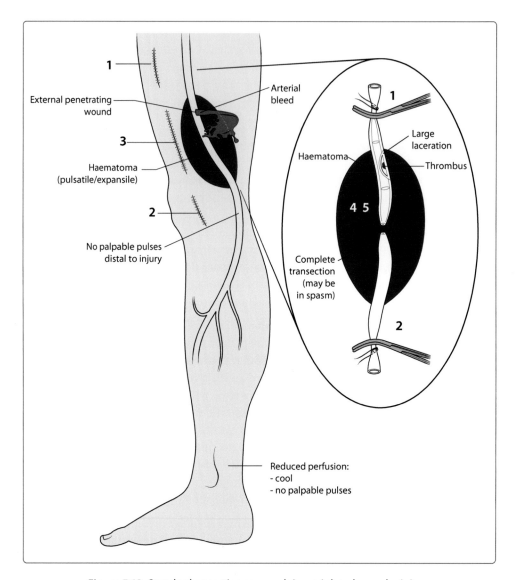

Figure 5.12 Standard operative approach in peripheral vascular injury.

A. Control the haemorrhage
  1. Proximal control first
  2. Distal control
  3. Open the haematoma and visualise the injury
B. Manage ischaemia
  4. Shunt the vessel across the injury if physiologically unwell or there are multiple competing injuries
  5. More definitive repair if physiology/time allows
     Vein graft from the contralateral (uninjured) limb
     Synthetic graft
C. Perform a fasciotomy

concurrent injuries. Although vein grafting is associated with better resistance to infection in elective vascular practice, this has not been well supported in the trauma literature, with similar rates of infection reported between vein and prosthesis (<2%). Of note however, infected venous grafts (in any situation) are prone to autodigestion after infection and rapid bleeding from a 'blowout', compared with synthetic grafts which have a tendency to form a pseudoaneurysm. Provision of good muscle and tissue cover over a vascular repair is most important to reduce infection risk, regardless of the choice of repair.

Shunting vascular injuries

Shunts may be inserted into any large vessel including the carotid, aorta, iliac arteries, mesenteric arteries and IVC, but the technique is particularly useful in peripheral vascular injury especially in the presence of a co-existing skeletal or soft tissue injury where rapid reperfusion is preferable prior to further management of other injuries (**Figure 5.7**). The shunt may be fixed *in situ* with ligatures and left until skeletal fixation is achieved and subsequently removed for definitive vascular repair, as appropriate. Alternatively, in the exsanguinating patient, a shunt may be inserted and firmly tied *in situ* as a damage control measure. Although it is desirable to remove the shunt within 6–12 hours, this decision is determined by patient physiology and metabolic derangement. Shunts have reportedly been left *in situ* for longer, without anticoagulation whilst awaiting reversal of the triad of death with no increase in mortality or morbidity. In general, if an injured limb is shunted as part of the damage control sequence, then fasciotomies should be performed distally as an adjunct to optimal limb perfusion (see later). A venous injury may also be shunted to mitigate against the swelling and vascular ooze expected after a dual arterial-venous injury due to the acute venous hypertension seen with acute venous ligation (**Figure 5.13**).

Tips for vessel shunting

- Do not have too much shunt upstream or downstream
  - Greater resistance to flow and risk of thrombosis
- Aim for the right amount of shunt coiling (redundancy) outside of the vessels
  - If too much then there will be greater resistance to flow and higher thrombosis risk
  - If too short there is a risk of the shunt falling out, especially with bony manipulation
- Aim to shunt the injured vein also
  - Greater arterial shunt patency
  - Less limb oedema
  - Greater chance of limb salvage
  - Less bleeding from limb acutely
  - Less venous hypertension in limb

The neck and thoracic outlet

The vascular structures in the neck and thoracic outlet account for <2% of all vascular trauma but are associated with a very high mortality and morbidity (including stroke). Vessels include the carotid and subclavian arteries and may be either *penetrating or blunt* , The prevalence of a significant vascular injury here is about 20% for stab wounds and 35% for

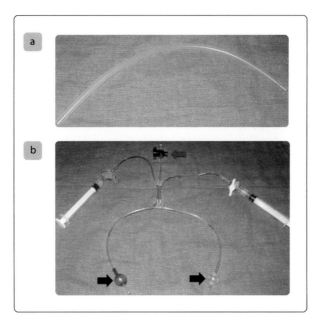

Figure 5.13 Commercially available vascular shunts licenced for carotid surgery usage. (a) Javid shunt, (b) Pruitt-Inahara shunt (arrows showing the inflated balloons used to keep the shunt *in situ*). In reality, any wide bore sterile plastic tubing may be used as a peripheral vascular shunt.

gunshot wounds (GSWs) with an historical intervention rate of 10% and 20% respectively. Blunt vascular injury is much less common, but is associated with a much higher incidence of stroke and TBI. Vascular injuries (especially penetrating) are best described in terms of 'zones of the neck' (**Figure 5.14**).

Physical examination alerts the trauma surgeon to the likely zone of injury, but caution is advised, as *injuries often involve more than one zone* (especially penetrating as the trajectory of the penetrating missile may cross the zonal boundaries or even other body cavities regardless of surface wound position. Always assume that the missile has violated more than one zone or region and prepare accordingly. **Figure 5.15** illustrates the close association and arrangement of the major vessels in the neck and chest, especially if the injury involves the thoracic outlet (i.e. zone I of the neck).

Trajectory determines injury

Penetrating missiles (especially gunshot wounds) do not respect anatomical boundaries

Pre-hospital and emergency management

Blunt vascular injury in the head and neck is typically associated with multiple competing injuries (e.g. TBI, spinal cord injury), which may require more urgent treatment first. Decide

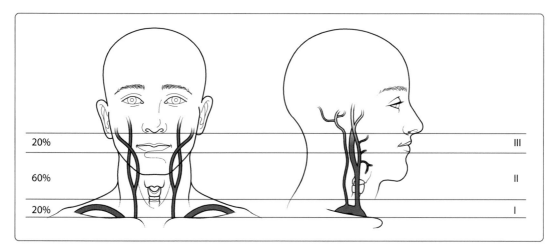

Figure 5.14 Zones of the neck and percentage involvement in penetrating injuries. Zone I: From the level of the clavicles to the cricoid cartilage and contains the subclavian vessels and common carotid artery and V1 of the vertebral artery. Zone II: From the cricoid cartilage to the angle of the mandible and contains the common carotid artery and bifurcation, the internal jugular vein, vagus nerve and V2 of the vertebral artery. Zone III: From the angle of the mandible to the base of the skull and contains the internal carotid artery and V3 of the vertebral artery.

early if the patient requires immediate surgical intervention versus further diagnostic workup. Perform RSI early and pre-emptively if there are concerns regarding airway compromise or the predicted clinical course is one of decompensation or airway demise. Use fluids sparingly (especially with penetrating injury) and employ *hypotensive resuscitation* as a workup for intervention and haemostasis. External active bleeding may be managed with direct pressure.

The neck is a semi-compressible region; although direct compression may be applied to the area bleeding, the airway and blood supply to the brain must not be compromised from the pressure. Also, the hard signs of vascular injury may be difficult to recognise in the neck. Certainly, an expanding or pulsatile haematoma or a thrill/bruit may be appreciated, but the loss of a distal pulse cannot be reliably examined for.

Diagnostic workup and investigations

Emergency management of penetrating neck injury (PNI)
- Perform plain x-ray (with skin markers)
  - Chest
  - Neck
  - Head
- Manage bleeding with pressure
  - Foley catheter counter-traction may be used in zone I injuries with variable effect
- Wound explorations should only take place in the operating room
- Administer anti-tetanus

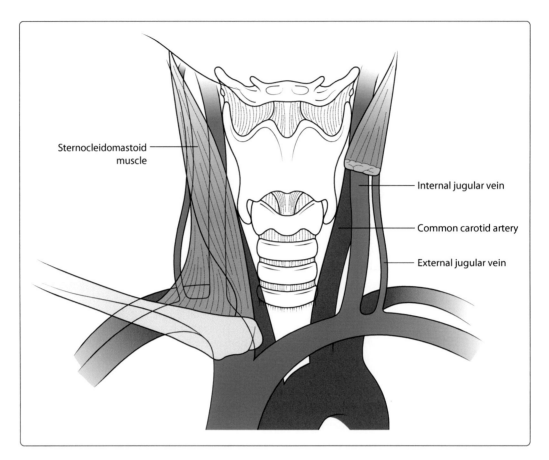

Figure 5.15 Gross anatomy of the carotid artery. The carotid sheath (carotid complex, internal jugular vein (IJV) and vagus nerve) lies behind the sternocleidomastoid muscle and is approached *via* a long incision just in front of the anterior border of this muscle. The muscle is then retracted in a posterior direction, exposing the carotid sheath, with the IJV lying in front of the other structures. The facial vein (branch leaving the anterior IJV) is the gatekeeper to the carotid bifurcation and must be ligated and divided, allowing the IJV to be retracted in a posterior direction. This, in turn, exposes the common carotid artery and its bifurcation into the external and internal carotid arteries medial and lateral, respectively. In addition, the internal carotid artery is recognised as having no branches in the neck. In addition, this illustration shows the root of the vessels coming off the aortic arch, below the clavicles (very challenging to access).

Clinical examination

Clinical examination has a reported accuracy of 70%–100% in the literature (most accurate in the awake patient with a zone II injury) to clinically rule out a significant vascular injury. However, in the *haemodynamically unwell patient, operative management is mandatory and assume all zones are involved.*

Plain x-ray

X-ray the neck in all penetrating injuries to look for foreign bodies (e.g. bullet) and use skin markers over the wound(s) to predict trajectory. Perform a chest x-ray (CXR), as 10%–15% will have a concomitant pneumothorax. Suspect phrenic nerve injury if an elevated hemi-diaphragm is seen, whereas a widened superior mediastinum (i.e. higher than where the

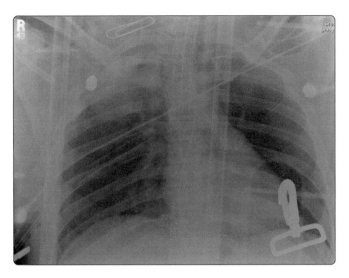

Figure 5.16 CXR showing a right-sided supraclavicular wound (paperclip) and a bullet lodged in the upper right lung. There is also a fractured right 1st and 2nd ribs, a right-sided pneumothorax (with chest drain *in situ*). The patient is also intubated with an NG tube *in situ*.

wide mediastinum is normally seen with traumatic aortic transection) is often associated with brachiocephalic (innominate) arterial injury (**Figure 5.16**).

Computed tomography (CT) angiography

CT angiography is the most sensitive investigation and is performed in all physiologically well patients for both trajectory determination (penetrating injury) and injury identification. CT scanning is less sensitive for stab wounds (low energy imparted into tissues) but will identify significant vascular injury (arterial contrast phase). Other neck structures are also visualised, including haematoma and its proximity to vascular structures. In the presence of metallic foreign bodies (e.g. shotgun injury), scatter from the pellets (shot) may decrease the accuracy of the imaging.

Arch angiography and four vessel angiogram

Despite being the gold standard of imaging, this is typically reserved for patients undergoing a radiological therapeutic intervention, after the injury has been identified on another modality. Drawbacks include arterial plaque giving a false positive result and it does not visualise other non-vascular neck structures.

Arterial duplex

An arterial duplex is a safe, reliable, repeatable, non-invasive bedside test. It may be useful for zone II injuries, but it does not visualise zones I or III injuries effectively or if the patient has an obese neck. It is often not available out of hours and is very user-dependent. Penetrating trauma with subcutaneous emphysema will generate poor acoustic windows in the tissues, thereby reducing accuracy and may be very painful to image against the skin in the awake patient.

Blunt carotid injury

Blunt carotid injuries carry a high mortality and stroke rate. Unfortunately, many patients also have a concomitant significant TBI, accounting for the high mortality and poor neurological outcomes. In addition, patients often present with multiple other competing injuries including chest, abdomen and pelvis, contributing to mortality. If the patient is physiologically well enough with no immediate indication for surgery, then an arterial and venous phase contrast CT scan (head to pelvis) is the diagnostic test of choice in blunt neck trauma. *Table 5.4* outlines the described grade of vessel injury and its associated mortality and stroke rate. Often the neurological injury has already occurred at the time of presentation (head trauma and embolic stroke), which determines the final outcome for the patient rather than any direct intervention that the surgeon can offer.

Management

Unfortunately, irreversible neurological damage has typically already occurred at the time of injury from either associated TBI, high spinal cord or embolic stroke from vessel injury itself. Unfortunately, surgery has not been shown to alter either the mortality or stroke rates in these patients although free haemorrhage should undergo surgical intervention (but mortality approaches 100% in this subset).

Only therapeutic anti-coagulation (heparin or low molecular weight heparin) has demonstrated any survival or stroke benefit for these patients. Unfortunately, anticoagulation is often contraindicated in the acute stages of polytrauma, especially when TBI or SCI is present. Free haemorrhage mandates immediate operative management but may not alter the outcome (100% mortality in the largest historical series). Endovascular intervention as an alternative to surgery may have a role in selective cases, but this has not been well scrutinized

Table 5.4 Carotid and vertebral artery injury grade and associated stroke rate and mortality

Injury grade	Abbreviated injury score (AIS)		Stroke rate (%)		Mortality (%)		Description
	Intracranial	Extracranial	Carotid	Vertebral	Carotid	Vertebral	
I	3	3	3	19	11	31	Intimal tear or dissection <25% luminal narrowing
II	3	3	11	40	11	0	Intimal tear, dissection, wall haematoma or luminal thrombus >25% luminal narrowing
III	3	3	33	13	11	13	Pseudoaneurysm
IV	4	3	44	33	22	11	Occlusion
V	5	4	100		100		Transection with free haemorrhage

Source: Adapted from Biffl WL et al., *J Trauma* 1999;228:462–479.

Table 5.5 Indications for Operative Exploration

1. Hard signs of vascular injury
2. Dysphonia or voice change
3. Haemoptysis, dysphagia or odynophagia
4. Haematemesis

to date in the trauma literature. A post-hanging injury, although by definition 'blunt', should be repaired if grade 2 or greater, especially in the absence of neurology. A grade 1 injury may be managed with simple observation and an anti-platelet agent (e.g. aspirin).

Penetrating carotid injury

Many penetrating neck injuries (PNIs) are managed non-operatively on a selective basis, but indications for immediate exploration are summarised in *Table 5.5*. *Always have a low threshold for exploratory surgery.*

Surgical management has more to offer PNI's compared with blunt injuries, and most decisions can be made on clinical grounds alone (but a pre-operative CT angiogram can also yield useful information if patient physiology allows).

> All haemodynamically unwell patients or those with hard signs of vascular injury must undergo immediate operative exploration and control

Principles of operative management of vascular injuries to the neck

- **Wide exposure**
  - Prepare chest and neck for surgery from xiphisternum to ear
  - Assume all zones are involved
- Proximal and distal control above and below the site of injury
  - Get proximal control for a zone I injury form within the chest
- **Shunt**
  - If prolonged surgery planned
  - If internal carotid artery (ICA) involved
- **Repair**
  - Primary repair (if tension-free)
  - Patch repair (if anterior wall only involved)
  - Interposition graft (to reconstruct injured segment)
- **Ligation**
  - If *in extremis*
  - Stroke rate 15%–20%
- **High zone III injury (uncontrollable/non-reconstructable)**
  - Insert a Fogarty balloon into the vessel, inflate, clip and cut
  - Ligate proximal segment (but try to keep external carotid artery [ECA] in circuit)
- **Other injuries**
  - Place a muscle patch between vascular and aerodigestive repairs

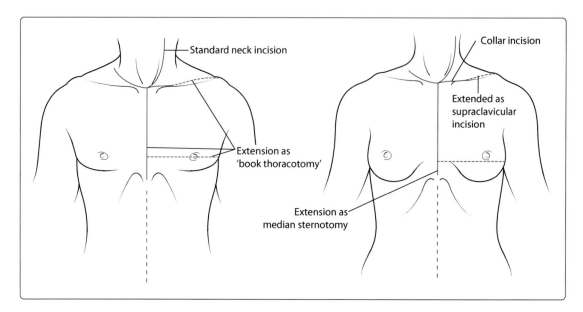

Figure 5.17 Approaches for control of the vessels in the neck and thoracic outlet.

Early airway control (RSI) is preferable if there are any concerns for an evolving airway complication. Always prepare the leg for harvesting long saphenous vein (LSV). All patients undergoing surgery must have the thorax prepared within the operative field in case proximal control needs to be achieved from inside the chest. Although a zone II carotid injury is the most common injury, injuries in zones 1 and 3 are particularly challenging (**Figure 5.17**).

Zone II injury

Zone II is the most frequently injured zone stretching from the *cricoid cartilage to the angle of the mandible*, housing the structures of the anterior triangle of the neck (**Figure 5.18**). Zone II injuries are exposed *via* the standard 'carotid surgery' exposure as a generous longitudinal incision along the anterior border of the sternocleidomastoid muscle (SCM), dividing skin, subcutaneous tissue and platysma muscle. Expect haematoma along the way within the tissue planes. Retract SCM backwards (posterior direction) to expose the internal jugular vein (IJV). The external jugular if encountered is ligated. The facial vein must be identified as it joins the anterior border of IJV as this is the 'gatekeeper' to the carotid complex (typically straddles the level of the carotid bifurcation), which also typically lies just proximal to the angle of the mandible. Ligate and divide the facial vein to allow retraction of the IJV backwards. It is best to dissect the common carotid proximal (lower down) in the neck first to get proximal control (and it is easier to dissect here with less additional anatomical structures).

If a carotid injury is present, adventitial disruption and haematoma (often small) will be visible. If so, the interior of the vessel must also be inspected no matter how innocuous or haemostatic the exterior of the vessel looks, as simple perforations may hide a more extensive injury such as an intimal tear and thrombus (**Figure 5.19**).

Once vessel control (looping and clamping) is achieved, a longitudinal arteriotomy is performed along the vessel until normal, to visualise the inside of the vessel. Injured

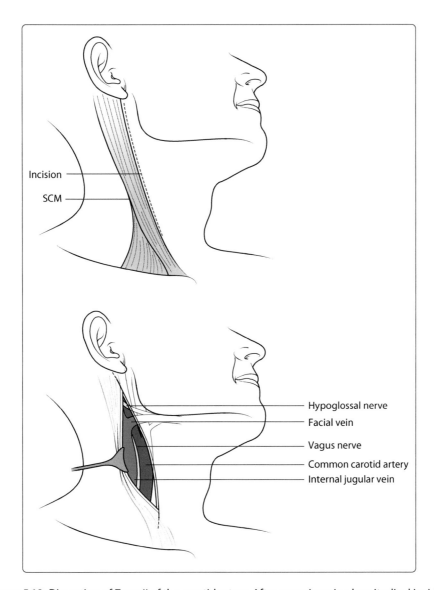

Figure 5.18 Dissection of Zone II of the carotid artery. After exposing *via* a longitudinal incision along the anterior border of sternocleidomastoid muscle which is subsequently retracted backwards, the carotid sheath is exposed. The IJV lies in front and anterior to the carotid artery. The facial vein (typically overlying the carotid bifurcation) is ligated and divided, thereby allowing backward retraction of the IJV with exposure of the common, external and internal carotid arteries.

intima may be directly repaired (if not ragged) or resected (akin to an endarterectomy) back to healthy, injury-free tightly adherent intima, before repair of the vessel. A carotid shunt should be used if surgery is prolonged (**Figures 5.20 and 5.21**).

The carotid may be amenable to direct repair with an end-to-end anastomosis, but only if tension-free. Otherwise an interposition graft (vein or synthetic) may be used. If vein is used, do not physically (anatomically) reverse it (**Figure 5.22**). The venous valves need to allow blood flow antegrade and unobstructed towards the brain. If only the anterior wall is injured (unlikely), then a patch graft repair may be performed. Always explore for

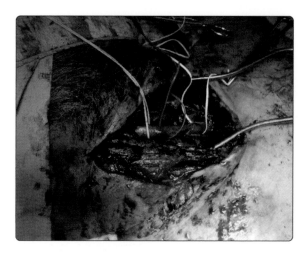

Figure 5.19 Shotgun injury to the right neck. The common carotid artery is exposed and looped. There are multiple bruises on the anterior carotid surface from the injury. The inside of the carotid will require surgical exploration.

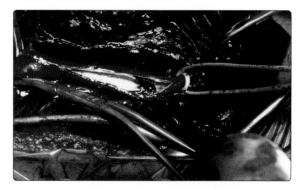

Figure 5.20 Looped and clamped right common carotid artery after stabbing. Thrombus and injured intima are visible, which were removed. The back wall was only held by a thin layer of adventitia and could not be safely repaired primarily.

a concomitant aerodigestive injury, and if present, repair with an interposition muscle patch to protect the vascular anastomosis from infection and blowout (usually fatal).

Alternatively, for the patient *in extremis*, the vessel may be ligated, but there is a risk of acute stroke. Acute ligation of the common carotid artery (CCA) is associated with an acute stroke rate of 15%–20% in the literature, although this may be as high as 40%–50% if the ICA is ligated or in the shocked severely injured patient.

The use of covered stents placed in IR has been described with good success, but many of these injuries will require open surgery anyway, due to other concomitant injuries and the high incidence of severe haemorrhage mandating immediate surgical control. Also, if thrombus is present in the lumen of the carotid, IR may dislodge this leading to acute stroke.

Zone I neck injuries start in the *thoracic outlet* extending from the *clavicles* to the level of the *cricoid cartilage*. Access here is very challenging. A small contained haematoma within zone I may occasionally be managed by IR with a covered stent if

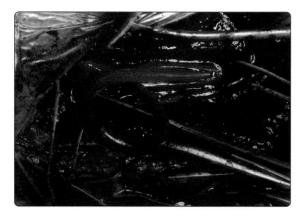

Figure 5.21 Javid shunt inserted in the CCA while the LSV was harvested for interposition grafting. The patient was physiologically well enough for definitive repair. Otherwise, the shunt could have been left *in situ* pending reversal of the metabolic derangement.

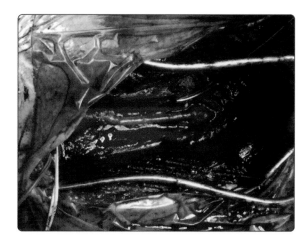

Figure 5.22 LSV interposition grafting (vein not anatomically reversed) of the CCA.

haemodynamically well enough. However, zone I injuries cannot be controlled safely through a neck dissection alone and therefore proximal control is obtained from inside the chest either *via* median sternotomy (preferable) or clamshell thoracotomy (*in extremis*). The proximal brachiocephalic (innominate), left CCA and left subclavian artery (SCA) are safely controlled within the chest (as appropriate), although accessing the left SCA is difficult with a median sternotomy due to its deep posterior position at origin along the aortic arch (orientated anterior to posterior rather than a right-to-left direction). The left SCA may be more amenable to access and control through a 5th intercostal space left lateral thoracotomy or even a high left lateral thoracotomy *via* the 2nd or 3rd intercostal space. If the patient is *in extremis*, then a clamshell thoracotomy is appropriate which gives excellent exposure of the heart, aorta, aortic arch and its great branches (**Figure 5.23**).

If a median sternotomy has been performed, the incision may be extended further cephalad (into the neck) along the anterior border of the SCM (as described earlier) for a concomitant

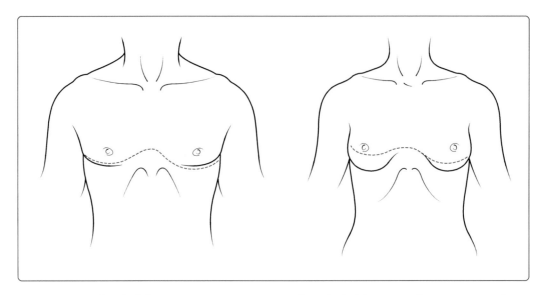

Figure 5.23 Clamshell thoracotomy. It is important to place the incision across the sternum, not the xiphoid. Placing the incision too inferiorly will hamper exposure.

zone II carotid injury or extended laterally at the top end along the superior border of the clavicle (collar incision) for a concomitant SCA injury (**Figures 5.24 and 5.25**). The old fashioned 'trap-door' incision consisting of a supraclavicular dissection, upper median sternotomy and high anterior anterolateral thoracotomy on the same side to allow the anterior chest to be partially opened is a difficult and cumbersome to perform technique, that leaves a morbid, painful wound, and offers no exposure advantage over the approaches described

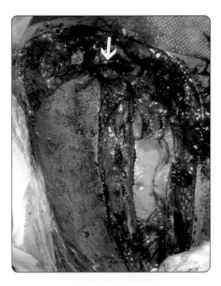

Figure 5.24 Right SCA injury from GSW. This has been controlled proximally using a median sternotomy and extended laterally in the supraclavicular fossa. A shunt (arrow) has been inserted to control haemorrhage and maintain right upper limb perfusion. Once physiologically well, the patient was returned to theatre for venous interposition grafting (reversed vein).

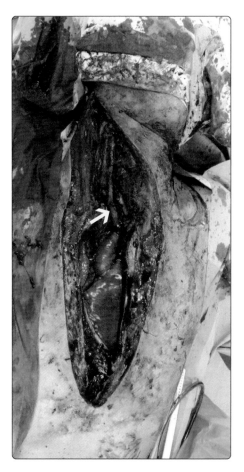

Figure 5.25 Proximal control of a zone I injury (GSW) *via* a median sternotomy. The incision was extended cephalad to expose the carotid arterial complex. The injury visualised involves the brachiocephalic artery (arrow).

earlier. It is therefore no longer recommended. Clamping of an injured great vessel may be performed close to or even partially occluding the aortic arch at origin (side-biting Satinsky clamp, **Figure 5.26**). The vessel may be repaired directly or with an interposition graft. If badly injured, it may need to be ligated and a non-anatomical bypass performed. Intimal injuries with acute thrombosis may be managed with thrombectomy and direct repair.

Zone III injury

Zone III extends from the angle of the mandible to the base of the skull (BOS) with a narrow conical configuration (carotid siphon), as it ascends towards the BOS. Access is further limited by the BOS itself, the mastoid bone and styloid process, making this area a challenging space for surgical access. In addition, distal control of a carotid injury in zone 3 is almost impossible to achieve. If possible, manage with IR and a covered stent or occasionally with an occlusion device. Small pseudoaneurysms of the ICA may be observed with surveillance CT angiography as many will heal over time.

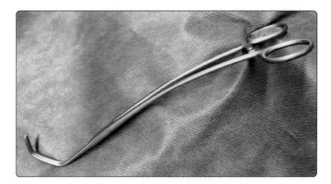

Figure 5.26 Satinsky clamp. This is a hockey-stick-shaped vascular clamp that may be used to completely occlude a vessel or in a side-biting fashion to partially occlude.

Table 5.6 Surgical options to gain control of a difficult zone III vascular injury

Technique	Drawback
• Open mouth wide	• Sterility may be compromised, difficult to maintain
• Dislocate mandible forwards	• Difficult to maintain without wires
• Mandibular osteotomy	• Difficult to perform and time-consuming
• Mastoidectomy	• Difficult to perform and time-consuming
• Excision of jugulo-digastric muscle	• Hypoglossal nerve may be injured
• Excision of styloid bone	• Can be difficult to perform
• Mobilise external ear	• Cosmetic effect and sterility may be compromised
• Nasal intubation	• Dangerous unless performed pre-operatively
• Pass Fogarty balloon into vessel, inflate it and leave *in situ*	• Foreign body left *in situ*, stroke risk
• Apply two metal clips close to the balloon, cut the catheter and leave *in situ*	• Stroke risk 10%–20%
• Ligate it and leave it!	

Zone III injuries are challenging because this distal segment of internal carotid artery is difficult to safely and rapidly access and looping and clamping is often not possible if the injury is very high. The surgical approach is the same as for zone II, although extended more cephalad. If distal bleeding is still problematic there are numerous techniques described to aid surgical exposure, many of which are cumbersome to achieve and time-consuming, especially in the presence of rapid bleeding (*Table 5.6*). Adjunctive techniques for exposure include resecting the mastoid bone (mastoidectomy), dislocating the mandible forward, carrying the incision behind the ear to bring the ear forward, resecting the styloid process bone, resecting the mandibular ramus and dividing the jugulo-digastric muscle which overrides the distal ICA. A more practical solution is occlusion of the internal carotid artery using a Fogarty balloon catheter by inserting the balloon, inflating it to gain haemostasis and maintain *in situ* (**Figure 5.27**). Once haemorrhage is controlled, the surgeon may then perform a safer, more technical dissection to assess the injury and potential repair. If however the injury is inaccessible or impossible to repair or the patient is *in extremis*, the Fogarty catheter may be clipped to keep the balloon inflated and then cut proximally to leave the balloon *in situ*, followed by ligation of the vessel and closure of the wound.

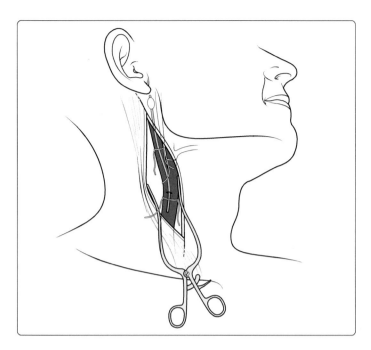

Figure 5.27 A Fogarty balloon catheter is inserted in a retrograde direction into the internal carotid artery to manage a high zone III carotid injury, that is inaccessible for repair or even ligation. The balloon is inflated to gain control of bleeding, after which the catheter is clipped (to prevent the balloon from deflating). If no other repairs are possible, cut the Fogarty proximal to this clip and leave the catheter and inflated balloon *in situ*.

Vertebral artery injuries

Trauma to the vertebral arteries (VAs) is rare, due to their deep and protected position within the neck, with rates slightly higher for penetrating over blunt trauma. There are four segments to the VA (V1 to V4) as described in **Figure 5.28**. V1 is the most frequently injured in penetrating injury but is very difficult to access as it is located in a medial position within zone I of the neck. V2 is well protected within the transverse processes of the C-spine but is challenging to expose when injured due its bony canal housing. V3 at the base of the skull posteriorly is almost inaccessible in an emergency and V4 can only be accessed with a posterior craniectomy. Many VA injuries will spontaneously thrombose, which may be managed expectantly. Small pseudoaneurysms may also be managed expectantly.

Due to the relative inaccessibility of these vessels, endovascular management is now considered the first line treatment with open repair reserved for failed endovascular repair with persistent active haemorrhage. The endovascular approach involves both antegrade travel from its SCA origin and retrograde (crossing the basilar artery from the contralateral side) to gain access to the vessel, typically followed by coiling (from both sides). The use of a covered stent is associated with a 100% thrombosis rate with an increased risk of posterior stroke.

Intraoperatively, a V1 injury (vertebral artery as is ascends from the subclavian artery before entering the bony canal at the level of C6) should be ligated, with little consequence. A V2 injury may be temporised by plugging the bony canal injury with bone wax to create a tamponading effect. Failure to achieve homeostasis will mandate

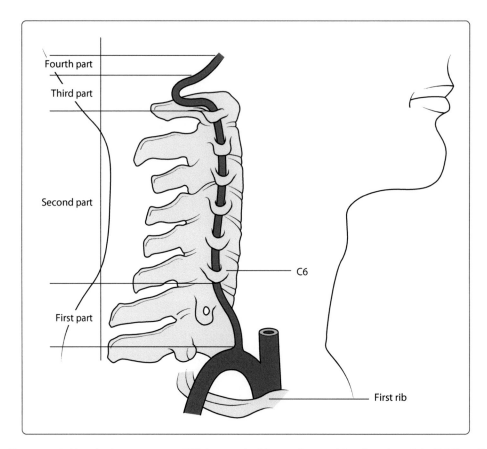

Figure 5.28 Vertebral artery course. VI is in zone I of the neck, stretching from its origin (SCA) until it enters the vertebral bony canal at the level of C6. V2 is within the bony vertebral canal (transverse processes) in zone II of the neck. V3 begins as it exits from the vertebral canal until entering the skull and V4 represents its intracranial portion.

direct surgical exposure of V2 by dissecting and sweeping the carotid artery posterior to gain access to the anterior midline cervical vertebrae. Further exposure involves dissection of the cervical periosteum from the midline and sweeping it off the vertebrae in a postero-lateral direction to expose the transverse processes followed by opening of the vertebral canal with bone nibblers. This is a difficult and time-consuming technique in the face of active haemorrhage. Bone wax haemostasis may then be re-attempted. Otherwise the vessel should be ligated, including the surrounding vertebral vein (often duplicate).

Subclavian artery (SCA) and axillary artery injury

The SCA lies just superior to the clavicle on surface anatomy and is divided into three segments by the overlying anterior scalene muscle (ASM). Open, surgical access is difficult and time-consuming, with numerous important structures within its vicinity, an IR approach is often preferable in selected groups of patients.

In the emergency setting, a penetrating wound to the SCA may be temporised by carefully inserting a Foley catheter into the wound track and gently advancing it (**Figure 5.29**). Inflate

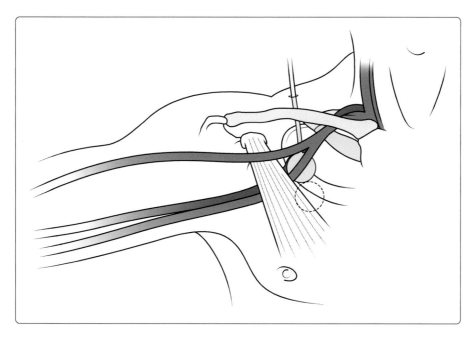

Figure 5.29 Foley Balloon counter-traction for zone I PNI with suspected SCA injury. The catheter is inserted carefully into the wound along the tract. Once inserted, the balloon is inflated and withdrawn to gain purchase against the bony clavicle. Theoretically, this will compress the injured vessel against the under surface of the clavicle.

the balloon and withdraw the catheter gently until the injured vessel is compressed up against the underside of the clavicle (or other tissue), thereby temporising the bleeding (**Figure 5.30**).

If a surgical approach is undertaken, the proximal SCA may require proximal control from within the chest (as in zone I injuries) (**Figures 5.31 and 5.32**). Distal control is obtained as a transverse incision for about 8–10 cm, from the midline and extending laterally, 1 cm (fingerbreadth) above the clavicle. After dissecting through skin, fascia and platysma, the clavicular insertion of sternocleidomastoid muscle (SCM) is divided

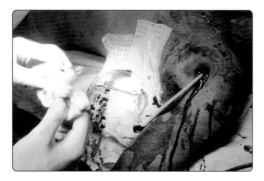

Figure 5.30 Foley catheter inserted along penetrating tract, and the balloon inflated and catheter withdrawn until resistance is felt. Note the clip at the top of the Foley catheter to stop blood coming out.

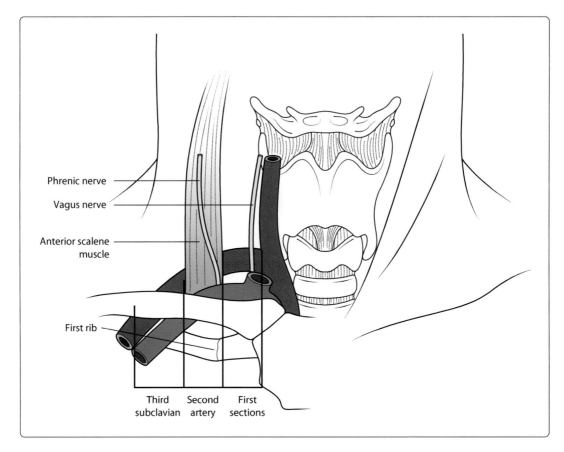

Figure 5.31 The subclavian artery (SCA) has three segments, with segment two covered by the anterior scalene muscle (ASM) and zones one and three proximal and distal to this respectively. The subclavian vein (SCV) lies in front of the ASM. The phrenic nerve travels within the anterior myofascia of the ASM in a lateral to medial (the only peripheral nerve to travel in a lateral to medial direction) direction and must be identified and protected during dissection. The ASM must be divided close to insertion to the first rib and dissected free to gain access to the SCA behind it.

(but preserve the sternal insertion). Once opened, the vascular fat pad is visualised. This is akin to muscle, as it is very vascular and should be preserved as it will serve as vascular tissue coverage after vessel repair. Mobilise it in a medial to lateral direction, but try not to divide completely (i.e. preserve it on a lateral pedicle of tissue, but reflected out of the surgical field). Once the fat pad is elevated, the SCV comes in to view, which is controlled and mobilised. Small injuries to the SCV may be sutured, but extensive injuries mandate acute ligation. The vein is retracted safely out of the field to reveal the ASM (**Figure 5.33**).

Once reflected, the ASM, with its phrenic nerve (often underwhelmingly small) is identified, passing on and within the thin fascial layer of the anterior surface of ASM. The phrenic nerve travels in a lateral-to-medial direction (the only peripheral nerve in the body to do so) and within the thin investing fascia on the anterior surface of the ASM. It is quite delicate and should be mobilised gently to avoid an ipsilateral diaphragmatic palsy.

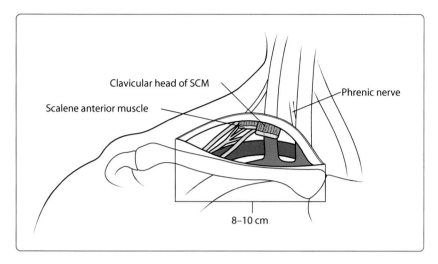

Figure 5.32 Supraclavicular subclavian artery (SCA) exposure. The SCA is approached by a transverse incision about I cm above and parallel to the clavicle starting over the clavicular head of SCM (which must be divided). It is divided into three segments by the anterior scalene muscle (ASM). The SCV lies in front of the ASM (but behind the scalene fat pad) and the phrenic nerve runs on its anterior surface within its fascia (the phrenic nerve is the only peripheral nerve that runs from lateral to medial) and must be protected. The ASM is carefully dissected off the to gain access to the SCA behind it. SCA1 is proximal to ASM, SCA2 lies behind it and SCA3 distal to it (before diving behind the clavicle).

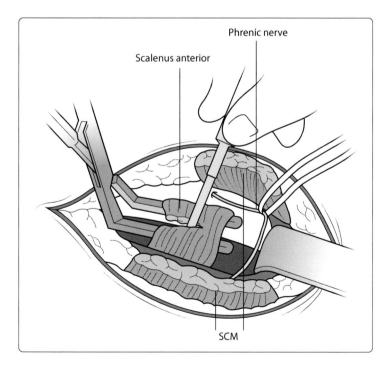

Figure 5.33 Once the scalene fat pad has been dissected free and the SCV retracted out of the surgical field, the ASM may be divided to gain access to the SCA directly posterior. While protecting the phrenic nerve with gentle retraction, divide the ASM (with electrocautery) close to insertion at the first rib.

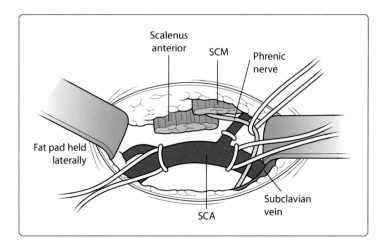

Figure 5.34 The ASM has been divided and allowed to retract upwards out of the surgical field. Segment 2 lies directly behind the ASM. Segments 1 and 3 have been looped for control.

It is the author's preference to loop the nerve gently so that it is identifiable in the field and may be mobilised (carefully) as required. Posterior to the ASM lies the middle scalene muscle (MSM) with the accompanying brachial plexus, which may interdigitate with fibres from the MSM. The SCA lies in between both of these scalene muscles. The proximal SCA (SCA1) is looped and controlled. With the phrenic nerve protected, divide the ASM close to its insertion into the first rib and allow it to retract upwards. This will then bring the SCA in to view (the second portion of the SCA lies behind the ASM [**Figure 5.33**]). Do not dissect any deeper lest a brachial plexus injury may occur. In addition, inspect for a brachial plexus injury as this is highly prevalent with an SCA injury (**Figure 5.34**).

The vessel is looped and controlled distally and the injured SCA assessed and repaired (or shunted) as appropriate. Repair may include direct suturing, interposition grafting or ligation and bypass grafting. However, access and space is very limited in this region of the neck and further dissection below the level of the clavicle may be required to manage complex injuries.

Therefore, SCA dissection may be combined with an *infraclavicular* (axillary artery) dissection as a combined supraclavicular–infraclavicular approach (joined as a lazy *S* across the clavicle). If the injury is behind the clavicle or access is still proving difficult, then the clavicle may be divided and removed as required. A tension-free direct anastomotic repair is typically not possible for injuries here and most will require interposition grafting. Shunting may be performed as part of DCS. Branches of the SCA (thyrocervical trunk, VA and internal thoracic [mammary] artery) may be ligated as required.

Internal jugular vein (IJV)

Simple injuries may be directly repaired, but if extensively injured, acute ligation should be performed which is typically without consequence (there is a theoretical risk of aggravating a raised intracranial pressure if there is concomitant TBI). Many repaired IJV's will thrombose after repair anyway. *Do not risk aggravating haemorrhage to try to salvage an already doomed IJV.* In addition, I do not recommend using the IJV as a venous patch due to its propensity to become aneurysmal over time and thrombose or rupture.

Axillary artery injury

The SCA becomes the axillary artery as it passes over the lateral border of the first rib underneath the clavicle. The axillary artery is divided into three anatomical segments by the presence of the overlying pectoralis minor muscle (overlies segment 2 of the axillary artery) (**Figure 5.35**). This is also the gatekeeper to the axillary artery and must be divided for complete exposure.

The best exposure is *via* a transverse incision for about 8–10 cm, 1 cm (fingerbreadth) below the clavicle starting at its medial 1/3 and extending outwards (almost a mirror image incision to the SCA exposure above, but more lateral). Once the skin, subcutaneous tissue and clavipectoral fascia is divided, the pectoralis major muscle is

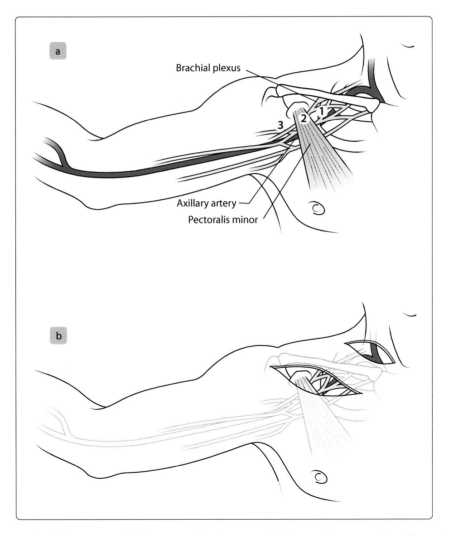

Figure 5.35 Axillary artery. (a) The pectoralis minor muscle is the gatekeeper to the axillary artery and is divided to gain access to the axillary artery and vein. The cords of the brachial plexus are intimately associated with the vessel and must be protected. (b) Axillary artery exposure. The axillary artery may be approached about 1cm below and parallel to the clavicle. With severe injury, proximal control may be approached above the clavicle at the SCA (as described earlier).

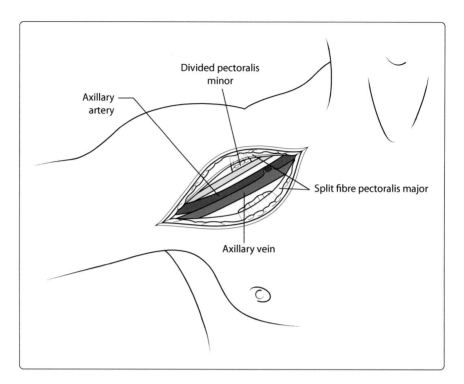

Figure 5.36 The fibres of the pectoralis major muscle are split (rather like a grid iron) to gain access to the pectoralis minor muscle (gate keeper to the axillary artery). This smaller muscle is encircled and divided with electrocautery. The axillary artery and vein (more anterior) and the cords of the brachial plexus are then identified.

opened in a muscle-splitting fashion. Alternatively, the pectoralis major muscle may be divided close to its tendinous insertion into the humerus and reflected out of the surgical field (leave enough cuff of muscle-tendon to repair afterwards) (**Figures 5.36 and 5.37**). The pectoralis minor muscle lies beneath and is encircled bluntly with a finger and haemostatically divided and is not repaired afterwards. This exposes segment 2 of the axillary artery and segment 1 and 3 may be dissected and controlled proximal and distal to this respectively.

The subclavian vein lies adherent (slightly antero-inferior) to the artery and may be duplicate or bifid. Also, the cords of the brachial plexus (lateral, posterior and anterior) surround the axillary artery here and must be identified (and inspected for trauma) and protected. The axillary artery injury may then be repaired directly or with an interposition graft as appropriate.

If injuries to the axillary artery are more extensive, it may be dissected and followed into the axilla, becoming the proximal brachial artery as it passes the lower border of terres major muscle. Care must be taken not to injure the numerous branches of the brachial plexus in this region (**Figure 5.38**).

Removal of the clavicle

As described earlier, for a combined SCA–axillary artery injury, or an injury occurring behind the clavicle, best exposure is with a combined SCA and axillary artery

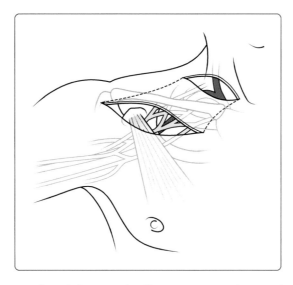

Figure 5.37 The incisions for subclavian and axillary exposure can be joined and the mid-clavicle removed to expose the anatomy *in continuum.*

dissection (**Figure 5.39**) followed by a claviculectomy. Use a periosteal elevator to separate any surrounding tissue, including the periosteum and the subclavius muscle (lies underneath the clavicle) from the bone. A bone cutter (or Gigli saw) is used both proximal and distal on the clavicle to remove as much of the middle portion of the bone as possible. Some authors have described dissecting the clavicle free at the clavi-sternal joint, but I feel that this is too cumbersome and time consuming to perform and unnecessary.

Once removed, this allows extensive exposure of the subclavian–axillary artery complex and any injuries may be safely managed.

Should the clavicle be replaced?   There is some evidence that leaving a patient without a clavicle leads to an unstable shoulder complex. Best evidence suggests that this will not interfere with normal daily activities, but only activities which stress the shoulder complex

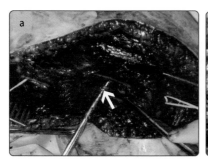
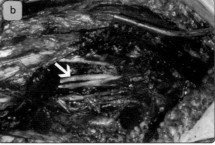

Figure 5.38 (a) Blunt injury to right axillary artery from anterior displacement of a comminuted humeral fracture, with severe contusion and occlusion of the vessel (arrow) (hard signs = loss of pulses in limb). (b) Interposition reversed vein graft repair (arrow) with restoration of perfusion.

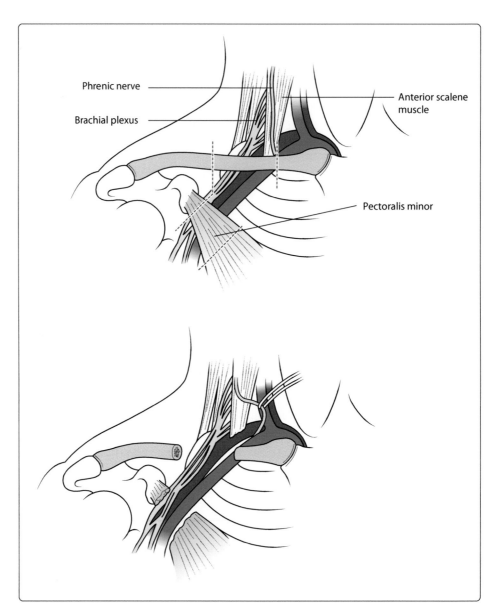

Figure 5.39 Once proximal SCA dissection and control (division of anterior scalene muscle) and distal axillary artery dissection and control (division of the pectoralis muscle) have been achieved, join these two surgical exposure incision across the clavicle. Using a Gigli saw, remove the central segment of the clavicle to expose the vessel behind it. Note that the pectoralis major is not included in this illustration and the phrenic nerve is protected.

more aggressively (e.g. sports). Unfortunately, even with replacement of the clavicle, there is still a risk of shoulder instability, non-union, mal-union, osteomyelitis and further pain and morbidity from a replaced, plated clavicle, including thoracic outlet syndrome (painful neurogenic type or occlusive arterial and venous type). Therefore, we do not advocate replacing and repairing the clavicle after a claviculectomy. Reconstruction may be performed later if required.

Brachial artery and forearm artery exposure

The upper limb is more resistant to acute ischaemia in comparison to the lower limb (especially if the upper limb injury occurs distal to the origin of the profunda brachii deep branch) (**Figure 5.40**). Thus, an upper limb amputation after an ischaemic injury is unusual. However, the long-term consequences of a missed or delayed vascular injury can be very morbid and life-changing, even if amputation is not required including; upper limb claudication, painful ischaemic neuritis and ischaemic contracture (e.g. Volkmann's ischaemic contracture). This is even more important if the dominant arm has been injured; therefore, the presence of hard signs in the upper limb should be managed aggressively and in a timely manner. Common injury sites include the brachial artery (typical injury is punching a pane of glass!) and the axillary artery (beware the anterior displacement of head of humerus dislocation). Either the radial or ulnar arteries may be ligated as long as one or other remains in circuit to perfuse the hand.

Vascular injuries to the arm can typically be temporised with a combination of direct pressure, compression dressing and TK application. This is often all that is required for the non-specialist. The brachial artery is exposed through the natural 'groove' palpated at the medial aspect of the upper arm between the biceps anteriorly and triceps posteriorly (remember this natural anatomical space may be distorted in trauma due to tissue injury and haematoma). Make a longitudinal incision along this anatomical groove for about 10–15 cm. Divide skin, subcutaneous muscle and fascia. The brachial artery lies deep and, adjacent to the median nerve (often more obvious as it is thicker and more prominent). Take care not to confuse the nerve with the brachial artery. The brachial vein is adjacent to the artery and may be duplicate or bifid. The basilic vein lies deep in this region but typically more posterior. If the basilic vein is dissected, then the surgeon has gone too posterior (common mistake with this exposure). Typically, there will be no pulse in the

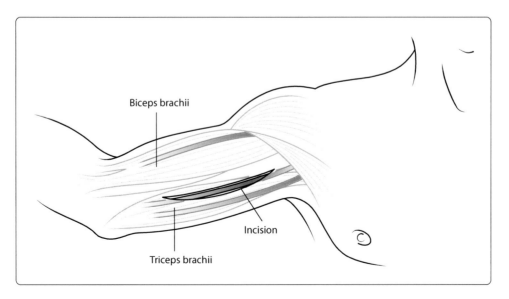

Figure 5.40 Brachial artery injuries are approached *via* a medial upper arm incision in the natural groove palpated between the biceps and triceps muscles.

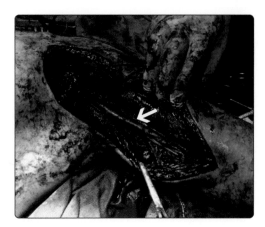

Figure 5.41 Interposition graft repair of left axillary and brachial artery (arrow).

injured brachial artery (thrombosis). Loop and control the vessel. Most brachial artery injuries will require an interposition graft or bypass with muscle cover, but the limb is quite resistant to ischaemia if ligation is required.

Once controlled, the brachial artery may be followed and dissected distally down the arm and into the forearm. It travels through the antecubital fossa and an *S*-shaped incision should be carried across the antecubital fossa (joint) here as it corresponds to the flexure surface of the elbow joint. Just beyond the antecubital fossa, it bifurcates into the radial and ulnar branches laterally and medially respectively (arm in the anatomical position). The interosseous branch may also be appreciated as it is typically large (**Figure 5.41**).

Peripheral vascular injury

Peripheral vascular injury is the most frequent type of vascular trauma encountered (>80% of vascular trauma) and is summarised in *Table 5.7*. *Table 5.8* summarises some classic trauma-vascular associations after blunt injury (these associations have a low sensitivity and are mainly historical) and a high index of suspicion is needed when patients present with one or more of these findings.

Physical examination

Most decision-making can be made on physical examination alone. This includes a detailed examination of the vascular, neurological, skeletal and soft tissues. Physical examination (hard signs of arterial injury) has been shown to be very reliable with a high degree of

Table 5.7 Aetiology of peripheral vascular injury

Penetrating	Gunshot, shotgun, stabbings, intravenous drug abuse
Blunt	Direct blunt injury (contusion), bony fracture, joint displacement
Iatrogenic	Arteriography, cardiac catheterisation, balloon angioplasty, inadvertent arterial puncture, aortic balloon pump

Table 5.8 Typical patterns of ortho-vascular trauma

Vascular injury patterns	
Injury mechanism	**Artery injury**
Posterior knee dislocation	Popliteal artery
Femur fracture	Superficial femoral artery
Supracondylar fractures	Brachial artery
Elbow dislocation	Brachial artery
Clavicular fracture	Subclavian artery
Anterior shoulder dislocation	Axillary artery

sensitivity (98%). In the presence of hard signs, immediate surgical exploration (without any further diagnostic workup) is mandatory.

In the absence of hard signs, significant vascular injury is unlikely and therefore operative exploration is unnecessary (unless other injuries require treatment). Further diagnostic workup is generally also unnecessary due to the very low incidence of significant arterial injuries in this group. All pulses must be palpated, both proximal and distal to the injury and comparison made with the contralateral (uninjured) limb. The approach to peripheral vascular injury is summarised in **Figure 5.42**.

Diagnostic studies

Diagnostic studies have not been shown to be superior over physical examination in ruling out a significant peripheral arterial injury

The absence of hard signs of vascular injury effectively excludes the presence of a significant arterial injury as reliably as any further diagnostic imaging

The presence of flow on a handheld Doppler device when used in isolation is not a reliable test of either the absence of vascular injury or adequate limb perfusion (**Figure 5.42**). A handheld Doppler is only useful if the ankle–brachial pressure index (ABPI) is also measured. The ABPI may be measured in the injured limb and compared with the contralateral (uninjured) limb. It is not reliable in the assessment of upper limb perfusion (due to the more ischaemia-resistant character of the arm). The normal ABPI is 0.9–1.1, which if present, effectively rules out a significant arterial injury with a very high negative predictive value. If ABPI <0.9, then a vascular injury is more likely. However, in the absence of hard signs, ABPI measurements offer little more in the assessment over physical examination alone. Therefore, if the ABPI is <0.9 in the absence of hard signs, it can typically be managed expectantly as any missed arterial injury is likely to

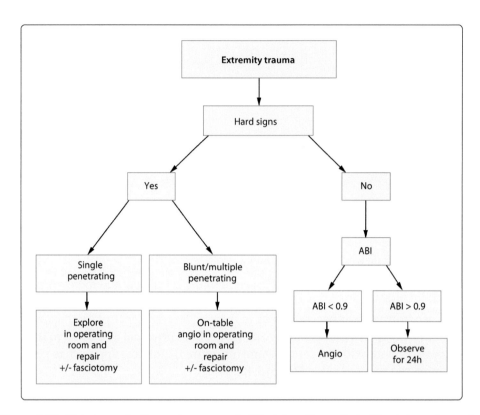

Figure 5.42 Clinical examination and assessment of the injured lower limb. If hard signs of vascular injury are present, then proceed to surgery. An on-table angiogram may be beneficial at the time of surgery, especially with blunt trauma where there may be more than one vascular injury. A fasciotomy must always be considered, depending on time to reperfusion and burden of injuries. If hard signs are not present or are equivocal, then significant malperfusion may be ruled out with an ABPI measurement.

be self-limiting (i.e. minimal vascular injury). Of course, this situation may evolve later into a complete arterial occlusion which will then mandate surgical management (but hard signs will also be present at this stage). Thus, the key to successful non-operative management in suspected peripheral vascular injury is serial physical examination, preferably by the same surgeon.

Vascular duplex is an accurate diagnostic test but is often unavailable out of normal working hours. A diagnostic angiogram with or without digital subtraction is still considered the gold standard diagnostic test in all vascular disease. However, it is only available in specialist centres, and unless the vascular injury is isolated and the patient physiologically well enough for transportation to the angiography suite, its use should be reserved for on-table angiography as an adjunct to operative management. Furthermore, as stated earlier, angiography has not been shown to be superior to physical examination alone in the assessment for significant arterial injury. CT scanning is now almost ubiquitous and has now all but replaced traditional catheter-directed (DSA) arteriography. It is a highly accurate diagnostic test, although minimal vascular injuries are also picked up frequently that do not require further treatment (**Figures 5.43 to 5.45**).

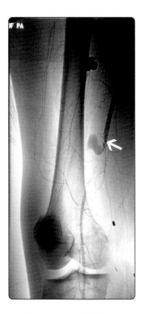

Figure 5.43 Angiogram of right lower limb post-GSW demonstrating occlusion of distal SFA with active bleeding (arrow).

> The presence of hard signs of vascular injury mandates surgical exploration

Operative management

In the absence of hard signs, patients may undergo further diagnostic workup or may be managed expectantly (non-operatively). The key to non-operative management is repeated and frequent physical examination such that should the situation evolve

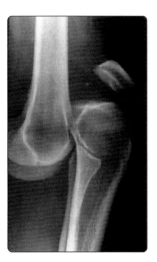
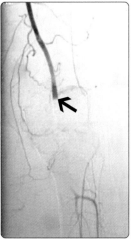

Figure 5.44 Posterior dislocation of the knee on plain x-ray. This patient had hard signs of vascular injury (i.e. loss of distal pulses). On-table angiogram demonstrated occlusion (arrow) of the popliteal artery secondary to an intimal flap.

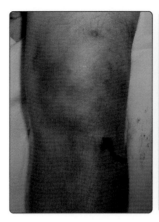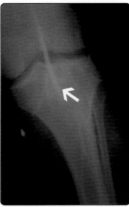

Figure 5.45 GSW with low velocity handgun to antero-lateral aspect, just below left knee joint. There were hard signs of vascular injury (absent pedal pulses). An on-table angiogram demonstrates a cut-off point (arrow) in the below-knee popliteal artery consistent with vessel injury. The bullet fragment is also seen medially.

(e.g. a non-occlusive injury progresses to an occlusive one), then surgical intervention will become necessary but without any demonstrable increase in morbidity in the literature.

When surgery is mandated, immediate transfer to the operating suite should take place. The massive transfusion protocol is initiated, as once the contained haematoma is opened, massive haemorrhage may occur. As with all vascular operations, proximal and distal control of the vessel occurs first (as described earlier) to minimise blood loss (*Table 5.9*). An on-table angiogram may be performed proximal to the injury if accurate location of the injured segment is warranted, but this is usually unnecessary and reserved for post-repair imaging only.

The segment of injured vessel may be resected and an interposition graft placed or it may be ligated followed by bypass (vein or synthetic graft). The recommended conduit of choice is a native (autologous) vein (preferably GSV), as many of these patients are young and fit and the longevity of a venous graft is better than synthetic. However, a synthetic graft may also be used to expedite limb reperfusion and earlier termination of surgery. If a autologous vein is used, then it is recommended to harvest from the contralateral (uninjured) limb. This is on the premise that, if the deep veins are also injured, then venous drainage will be more reliant on its superficial venous drainage

Table 5.9 Standard operative approach in peripheral vascular injury

1. Control the haemorrhage
   a. Proximal control first
   b. Distal control
   c. Open the haematoma and visualise the injury
2. Manage ischaemia
   a. Shunt the vessel across the injury if physiologically unwell or there are multiple competing injuries
   b. More definitive repair if physiology/time allows
      i. Vein graft from the contralateral (uninjured) limb
      ii. Synthetic graft
3. Perform a fasciotomy

alone and therefore the ipsilateral GSV should be preserved. Good tissue coverage (especially healthy muscle) is mandatory to avoid infection and graft 'blowout').

The junction zone of the pelvis with the lower limb

Injuries in this region are challenging, as there is a high prevalence of a concomitant injury within the pelvis as well as the proximal lower limb and groin. In addition, the vascular supply to the lower limb traverses the two adjacent zones here (junctional zone), and both the arterial and venous supply can lead to massive bleeding if injured with free haemorrhage into the pelvic cavity. Due to the anatomical constraints within this region, rapid control proximally is very challenging. TKs cannot be applied very proximal in the thigh. Furthermore, recognising the hard signs of vascular injury can be difficult if the injury is very proximal as it may be obscured by the pelvis (non-compressible cavity) (**Figure 5.46**).

Iliac vessel control

The external iliac artery (EIA) becomes the common femoral artery (CFA) as it passes under the inguinal ligament at the mid-inguinal point (halfway between the anterior superior iliac spine [ASIS] and the pubic symphysis). For proximal CFA or distal EIA injuries, the best and safest way to gain proximal control of the vessel is through an oblique (or wavy *S*) incision over the respective lower quadrant (i.e. pelvis). Incise through the skin and subcutaneous tissue until the external oblique fascia (external

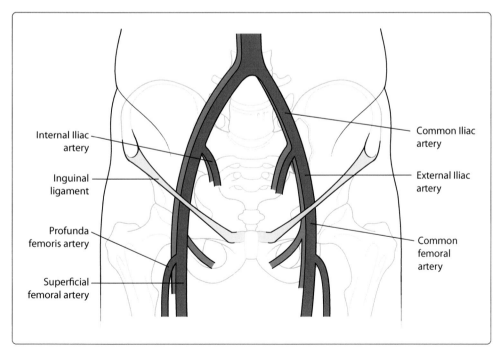

Figure 5.46 The junctional zone at the pelvis and proximal lower limb. The major vessels cross from the non-compressible pelvic cavity (the iliac vessels) into the lower limb (the external iliac artery becomes the common femoral artery as it passes underneath the inguinal ligament). It is difficult to obtain vessel control here without open surgical exposure.

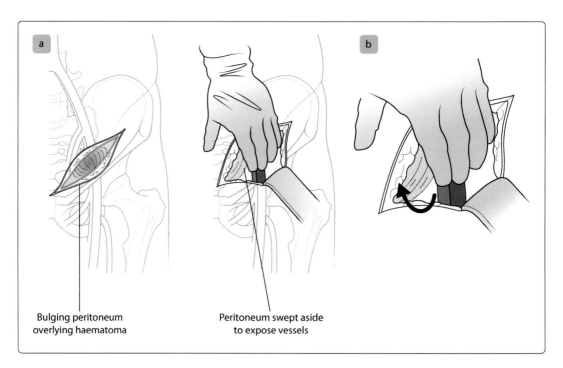

Bulging peritoneum
overlying haematoma

Peritoneum swept aside
to expose vessels

Figure 5.47 (a) An oblique incision over the lower quadrant, but parallel to and about 2 cm above the inguinal ligament is made. The external sheath is incised parallel to its fibres and the muscle of the anterior wall divided. (b) Once inside the true pelvis, the peritoneum is swept upwards away from the pelvis, revealing the iliac vessel underneath. If a haematoma is present, often the peritoneum will be dissected free from the pelvic side wall and the surgeon may enter this natural plane to control the vessels.

sheath) is reached. An oblique incision may then be made along its fibres (about 1–2 cm above its insertion to allow repair and approximation afterwards), straight through the entire anterior sheath (avoiding the rectus abdominis muscle medially) to gain direct access to the pelvic cavity.

The peritoneum overlying the pelvis (and separating it from the abdomen) is swept upwards and medially to expose the iliac vessel along the posterior pelvic wall. This is easier to do if there is a pelvic haematoma (as this auto-strips the peritoneum off the posterior wall of the pelvis), but if the injury is more distal and we are performing this manoeuvre to gain proximal vascular control, then the sweeping action is performed more vigorously by the surgeon's hand. The iliac vessel is then controlled and clamped as already described (**Figure 5.47**).

Femoral vessel dissection

The femoral vessels are exposed *via* a longitudinal incision in the groin over the mid-inguinal point. Make a 10–15 cm incision, dividing skin, subcutaneous tissue and the superficial and deep layers of fascia (**Figure 5.48**). This can be done more confidently if proximal control has already been obtained through the pelvis as described earlier. The gatekeeper here is the inguinal ligament, which must be exposed to visualise the CFA and to gain control. Take care to ligate the small inferior epigastric vein as it crosses anterior to the vessel (distal EIA) just under the inguinal ligament, which is easily injured and missed.

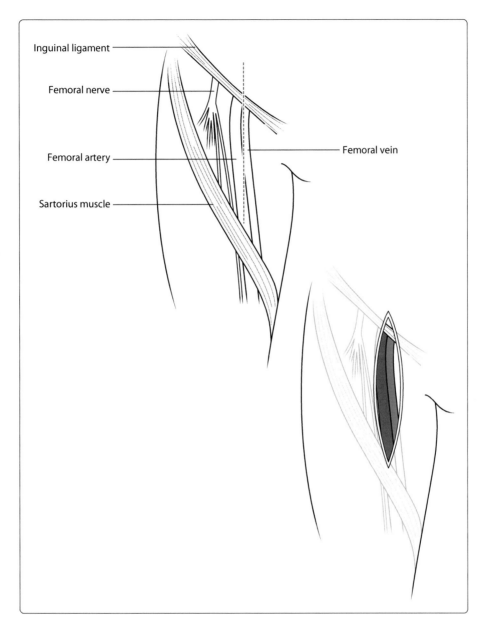

Figure 5.48 Common femoral artery exposure: A longitudinal incision is made well above the inguinal ligament and carried into the limb. The vessel as it passes under the inguinal ligament (external iliac artery becomes the common femoral artery at this point) is identified and controlled and then dissected further caudally to expose and control the superficial femoral artery and the profunda femoris artery.

If necessary, the inguinal ligament may be divided if rapid control is necessary, but must be repaired afterwards to avoid a pre-vascular hernia.

Follow the CFA distally to dissect and control the superficial femoral artery (now re-named the femoral artery) and the profunda femoris artery. Take care not to injure the femoral vein and its branches. In particular, the lateral circumflex femoral vein passes over the origin of the profunda femoris and is prone to injury and should be ligated.

Insert a vascular shunt and tie into position if haemodynamically unwell to maintain vessel continuity and prograde limb perfusion in addition to haemorrhage control. If there is a combined orthopaedic-vascular injury, it is important to establish adequate vascular perfusion before any other injuries are managed and a shunt is best used due to the high propensity for a vascular repair to become disrupted and thrombose during skeletal manipulation. Shunt insertion will re-establish flow allowing the other injuries to be managed before removing and performing the definitive repair (**Figures 5.49 and 5.50**).

Traditionally it was thought that an ischaemic limb had a 4–6 hour 'ischaemic window' before reperfusion needed to be reestablished to avoid permanent tissue injury. However, these figures apply to non-traumatised and non-shocked patients. The ischaemic window for the shocked, polytraumatised patient is much lower than for the acutely ischaemic, non-trauma patient. In addition, the original research into the ischaemic window times, pertained to the 'limb loss' rate only (rather than a good functional outcome rate). There is good clinical and animal based evidence, that in the shocked, polytraumatised patient, we should aim to reestablish perfusion of the injured limb (even with a shunt) within one hour of injury if a good, functioning limb is the

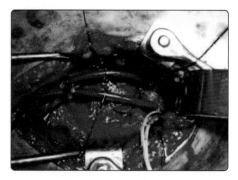

Figure 5.49 Shunting of both the femoral artery and vein. If possible, both vessels should be preserved and repaired. If a vessel has been shunted, then this must be documented with the date and time of surgery on the dressings if the patient is to be transferred out. In addition, leave TKs loosely applied for transfer in case of slippage of the shunt with massive haemorrhage. The distal limb must be left exposed to examine for perfusion in case of shunt thrombosis.

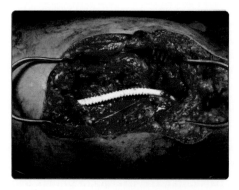

Figure 5.50 Repair of SFA using ring reinforced ePTFE after GSW to the thigh.

Table 5.10 Factors associated with high rates of limb loss in peripheral vascular injury

1. Treatment delay (>6 hours)
2. Shock
3. Blunt mechanism of injury
4. Lower extremity > upper extremity
5. Associated injuries
   a. Nerve (most predictive of amputation)
   b. Bone
   c. Vein
   d. Soft tissue
6. High velocity gunshot wound
7. Pre-existing disease (especially peripheral arterial disease)
8. Failure/delay in performing fasciotomy

desired primary outcome. Other factors associated with a higher limb loss rate are summarised in *Table 5.10*.

Venous injury

The combination of arterial and venous injury in a shocked patient is associated with an increased rate of amputation and poorer functional outcome (if limb loss does not occur). The management of venous injuries is somewhat controversial, especially in the presence of concomitant arterial injury. Injured deep veins may be either ligated or repaired (or shunted while awaiting repair). Although 30%–60% of venous repairs will occlude after about 2 weeks, we would recommend, where possible preserving venous flow (either shunt or repair) to reduce the acute venous hypertension and swelling that accompanies deep vein ligation. The reduction in the acute venous hypertension in the first few days is important for numerous reasons. It will minimise bleeding and the ongoing ooze that is seen after reperfusion (by reducing venous hypertension) especially if fasciotomies have also been performed, thus reducing blood loss and compartment syndrome as well as facilitating earlier closure of fasciotomy wounds with enhanced recovery, earlier ambulation and reduced hospital stay. By keeping the venous pressure close to normal will also reduce the limb loss rates after concomitant arterial repair, as well as improving the functional outcome for the patient by removing the risk of venous ischaemia in the limb while recovering from an ischaemia-reperfusion injury. A shunted or repaired vein is also associated with improved patency and longevity of an arterial shunt or repair respectively.

Furthermore, >50% of occluded venous repairs will re-canalize over time (with good long-term patency rates) thus helping to reduce chronic ambulatory venous hypertension and its long-term consequences. Thus, venous repair should be undertaken if possible, especially in the presence of a concomitant arterial-venous trauma, prolonged ischaemic time and significant blood loss with shock. This is especially important for popliteal arterial-venous injuries (much higher rate of limb loss). The vein may be repaired directly (unlikely) or with an interposition graft (non-reversed vein or synthetic). In the acute setting, both arterial and venous shunting should be performed pending definitive repair. Of course, if *in extremis*, then a venous injury may be ligated (although shunting and repair is still preferable if physiology allows) (**Figures 5.51 and 5.52**).

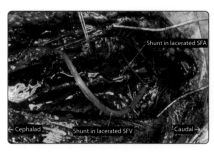 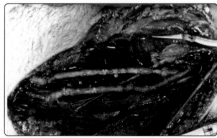

Figure 5.51 Figure showing shunt in both SFV and SFA after GSW to right groin (left) and with subsequent interposition vein repair of both artery (A) and vein (V) (right).

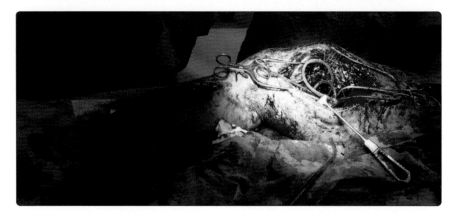

Figure 5.52 Fracture of right femur with SFA injury. A vascular shunt has been placed in the SFA to temporarily re-perfuse the lower limb to allow the orthopaedic surgeon manage the bony injury with external fixation. Calf fasciotomies have also been performed. The patient remained physiologically well and a definitive vascular repair was performed once bony fixation was complete.

Additional reading

Agarwal N, Shah PM, Class RH, Reynolds BM, Stahl WM. Experience with 115 civilian venous injuries. *J Trauma* 1982;22:827.

Applebaum R, Yellin AE, Weaver FA, Oberg J, Pentecost M. Role of routine arteriography in blunt lower extremity trauma. *Am J Surg* 1990;160:221–225.

Asensio JA, Britt LD, Borzotta A et al. Multiinstitutional experience with the management of superior mesenteric artery injuries. *J Am Coll Surg* 2001;193:354–365.

Asensio JA, Chahwan S, Hanpeter D et al. Operative management and outcome of 302 abdominal vascular injuries. *Am J Surg* 2000;180:528–533.

Attebery LR, Dennis JW, Russo-Alesi F, Menawat SS, Lenz BJ, Frykberg ER. Changing patterns of arterial injuries associated with fractures and dislocations. *J Am Coll Surg* 1996;183:377–383.

Berman SS, Schilling JD, McIntyre KE, Hunter GC, Bernhard VM. Shoelace technique for delayed primary closure of fasciotomies. *Am J Surg* 1994;167:435–436.

Biffl WL, Moore EE, Ellicott JP et al. The devastating potential of blunt vertebral arterial injuries. *Ann Surg* 2000;231:672–681.

Biffl WL, Moore EE, Offner PJ et al. Optimizing screening for blunt cerebrovascular injuries. *Am J Surg* 1999;178:517–522.

Biffl WL, Moore EE, Offner PJ, Brega KE, Franciose RJ, Burch JM. Blunt carotid arterial injuries: Implications of a new grading scale. *J Trauma* 1999;47:845–853.

Biffl WL, Moore EE, Ryu RK et al. The unrecognized epidemic of blunt carotid arterial injuries: Early diagnosis improves neurologic outcome. *Ann Surg* 1998;228:462–470.

Biffl WL, Ray CE, Moore EE, Mestek M, Johnson JL, Burch JM. Noninvasive diagnosis of blunt cerebrovascular injuries: A preliminary report. *J Trauma* 2002;53:850–856.

Boody AR, Wongworawat MD. Accuracy in the measurement of compartment pressures: A comparison of three commonly used devices. *J Bone Joint Surg Am* 2005;87:2415–2422.

Buckman RF, Pathak AS, Badellino MM, Bradley KM. Injuries of the inferior vena cava. *Surg Clin North Am* 2001;81:1431–1447.

Burch JM, Feliciano DV, Mattox KL, Bradley KM. Injuries of the inferior vena cava. *Am J Surg* 1988;156:548–552.

Caffarelli AD, Mallidi HR, Maggio PM, Spain DA, Miller DC, Mitchell RS. Early outcomes of deliberate nonoperative management for blunt thoracic aortic injuries in trauma. *J Thor Cardiovasc Surg* 2010;140:598–605.

Carrillo EH, Osborne DL, Spain DA, Miller FB, Senler SO, Richardson JD. Blunt carotid artery injuries: Difficulties with the diagnosis prior to neurologic event. *J Trauma* 1999;46:1120–1125.

Chambers LW, Green DJ, Sample K et al. Tactical surgical intervention with temporary shunting of peripheral vascular trauma sustained during operation Iraqi freedom: One unit's experience. *J Trauma* 2006;61:824–830.

Chirillo F, Totis O, Cavarzerani A. Usefulness of transthoracic and transesophageal echocardiography in recognition and management of cardiovascular injuries after blunt trauma. *Heart* 1996;75:301–306.

Clouse WD, Rasmussen TE, Peck MA et al. In-theatre management of vascular injury: 2 years of the Balad vascular registry. *J Am Coll Surg* 2007;204:625–632.

Cogbill TH, Moore EE, Jurkovich GJ, Feliciano DV, Morris JA, Mucha P. Severe hepatic trauma: A multi-center experience with 1,335 liver injuries. *J Trauma* 1988;28:1433–1438.

Davis TP, Feliciano DV, Rozycki GS et al. Results with abdominal vascular trauma in the modern era. *Am Surg* 2001;67:565–570.

de Mestral C, Dueck AD, Gomez D, Haas B, Nathens AB. Associated injuries, management and outcomes of blunt abdominal injury. *J Vasc Surg* 2012;56:656–660.

Demetriades D, Rabinowitz B, Pezikis A, Franklin J, Palexas G. Subclavian vascular injuries. *Br J Surg* 1987;74:1001–1003.

Demetriades D, Velmahos GC, Scalea TM et al. Diagnosis and treatment of blunt aortic injuries: Changing perspectives. *J Trauma* 2008;64:1415–1419.

Demetriades D, Velmahos GC, Scalea TM et al. Operative repair or endovascular stent graft in blunt traumatic thoracic aortic injuries: Results of an American Association for the Surgery of Trauma Multicenter Study. *J Trauma* 2008;64:561–571.

Dennis JW, Frykberg ER, Veldenz HC, Huffman S, Menawat SS. Validation of nonoperative management of occult vascular injuries and accuracy of physical examination alone in penetrating extremity trauma: 5 to 10 year follow-up. *J Trauma* 1998;44:243–253.

Dutton RP, Mackenzie CF, Scalea TM. Hypotensive resuscitation during active hemorrhage: Impact on in-hospital mortality. *J Trauma* 2002;52:1141–1146.

Dyer D, Moore E, Mestek M. Can chest CT be used to exclude aortic injury? *Radiology* 1999;213:195–202.

Fabian T, Devis K, Gavant M et al. Prospective study of blunt aortic injury. Helical CT is diagnostic and antihypertensive therapy reduces rupture. *Ann Surg* 1998;227:666–677.

Fabian TC, Patton JH Jr, Croce MA, Minard G, Kudsk KA, Pritchard FE. Blunt carotid injury: Importance of early diagnosis and anticoagulant therapy. *Ann Surg* 1996;223:513–525.

Feczko J, Lynch L, Pless J et al. An autopsy case review of 142 nonpenetrating (blunt) injuries of the aorta. *J Trauma* 1992;33:846–849.

Feliciano DV. Pitfalls in the management of peripheral vascular injuries. *TSACO* 2017;23:1–8.

Feliciano DV, Mattox KL, Graham JM, Bitondo CG. Five-year experience with PTFE grafts in vascular wounds. *J Trauma* 1985;25:71–82.

Frykberg ER. Advances in the diagnosis and management of extremity vascular trauma. *Surg Clin N America* 1995;75:207–223.

Frykberg ER, Crump JM, Dennis JW et al. Nonoperative observation of arterial intimal injuries in an experimantal model. *J Trauma* 1991;31:669–675.

Frykberg ER, Crump JM, Dennis JW, Vines FS, Alexander RH. Nonoperative observation of clinically occult arterial injuries: A prospective evaluation. *Surgery* 1991;109:85–91.

Frykberg ER, Dennis JW, Bishop K, Laneve L, Alexander RH. The reliability of physical examination in the evaluation of penetrating extremity trauma for vascular injury: Results at one year. *J Trauma* 1991;31:502–511.

Frykberg ER, Vines FS, Alexander RH. The natural history of clinically occult arterial injuries: A prospective evaluation. *J Trauma* 1989;29:577–583.

Giacobetti FB, Vaccaro AR, Bos-Giacobetti MA et al. Vertebral artery occlusion associated with cervical spine trauma: A prospective analysis. *Spine* 1997;22:188–192.

Gillespie DL, Woodson J, Kaufman J, Parker J, Greenfield A, Menzoian JO. Role of arteriography for blunt or penetrating injuries in proximity to major vascular structures: An evolution in management. *Ann Vasc Surg* 1993;7:145–149.

Granchi T, Schmittling Z, Vasquez J, Schreiber M, Wall M. Prolonged use of intraluminal arterial shunts without systemic anticoagulation. *Am J Surg* 2000;180:493–497.

Gulli B, Templeman D. Compartment syndrome of the lower extremity. *Orthop Clin North Am* 1994;25:677–684.

Hafez HM, Woolgar J, Robbs JV. Lower extremity arterial injury: Results of 550 cases and review of risk factors associated with limb loss. *J Vasc Surg* 2001;33:1212–1219.

Hansen CJ, Bernadas C, West MA et al. Abdominal vena caval injuries: Outcomes remain dismal. *Surgery* 2000;128:572–578.

Hargens AR, Schmidt DA, Evans KL et al. Quantitation of skeletal-muscle necrosis in a model compartment syndrome. *J Bone Joint Surg Am* 1981;63:631–636.

Ho R, Blackmore C, Bloch R. Can we rely on mediastinal widening on chest radiography to identify subjects with aortic injury? *Emerg Radiol* 2002;9:183–187.

Hobson RW, Yeager RA, Lynch TG et al. Femoral venous trauma: Techniques for surgical management and early results. *Am J Surg* 1983;146:220.

Hoffer EK, Sclafani SJ, Herkowitz MM, Scalea TM. Natural history of arterial injuries diagnosed with arteriography. *J Vasc Interv Radiol* 1997;8:43–53.

Kostler W, Strohm PC, Sudkamp NP. Acute compartment syndrome of the limb. *Injury* 2004;35:1221–1227.

Lebl DR, Dicker RA, Spain DA, Brundage SI. Dramatic shift in the primary management of traumatic thoracic aortic rupture. *Arch Surg* 2006;141:177–180.

Lee WA, Matsumura JS, Mitchell RS et al. Endovascular repair of traumatic thoracic aortic injury: Clinical practice guidelines of the society for vascular surgery. *J Vasc Surg* 2011;53:187–192.

Lim LT, Michuda MS, Flanagan P, Pankovich. Popliteal artery trauma: 31 consecutive cases. *Arch Surg* 1980;115:1307–1313.

Lin PH, Koffron AJ, Guske PJ et al. Penetrating injuries of the subclavian artery. *Am J Surg* 2003;185:580–584.

Loh SA, Rockman CB, Chung C et al. Existing trauma and critical care scoring systems underestimate mortality among vascular trauma patients. *J Vasc Surg* 2011;53:359–366.

Mathew S, Smith BP, Cannon JW, Reilly PM, Schwab CW, Seamon MJ. Temporary arterial shunts in damage control: Experience and outcomes. *J Trauma* 2017;82:512–217.

Mattox K, Feliciano D, Beal A. Five thousand seven hundred and sixty cardiovascular injuries in 4459 patients. Epidemiologic evolution 1958–1988. *Ann Surg* 1989;209:698–705.

McCready RA. Upper-extremity vascular injuries. *Surg Clin North Am* 1988;68:725–40.

Meyer J, Walsh J, Schuler J et al. The early fate of venous repair after civilian vascular trauma: A clinical, hemodynamic and venographic assessment. *Ann Surg* 1987;206:458.

Miller PR, Fabian TC, Croce MA et al. Prospective screening for blunt cerebrovascular injuries: Analysis of diagnostic modalities and outcomes. *Ann Surg* 2002;236:386–395.

Miranda FE, Dennis JW, Veldenz HC, Dovgan PS, Frykberg ER. Confirmation of the safety and accuracy of physical examination in the evaluation of knee dislocation for popliteal artery injury: A prospective study. *J Trauma* 2000;49:375.

Mirvis S, Bidwell J, Buddemeyer E et al. Value of chest radiography in excluding traumatic aortic rupture. *Radiology* 1987;163:487–493.

Mirvis S, Shanmugathan K, Miller B. Traumatic aortic injury: Diagnosis with contrast enhanced CT-five-year experience at a major trauma center. *Radiology* 1996;200:413–422.

Morrison CA, Carrick MM, Norman MA et al. Hypotensive resuscitation strategy reduces transfusion requirements and severe postoperative coagulopathy in trauma patients with hemorrhagic shock: Preliminary results of a randomized controlled trial. *J Trauma* 2011;70:652–663.

Murad MH, Rizvi AZ, Malgor R et al. Comparative effectiveness of the treatments for thoracic aortic transection. *J Vasc Surg* 2011;53:193–199.

Mwipatayi BP, Jeffery P, Beningfield SJ, Motale P, Tunnicliffe J, Navsaria PH. Management of extra-cranial vertebral artery injuries. *Eur J Vasc Endovasc Surg* 2004;27:157–162.

Neville RF, Hobson RW, Watanabe B et al. A prospective evaluation of arterial injuries in an experimental model. *J Trauma* 1991;31:669–675.

Nypaver TJ, Schuler JJ, McDonnel P et al. Long-term results of venous reconstruction after vascular trauma. *J Vasc Surg* 1992;16:762.

Panetta TF, Sales CM, Marin ML et al. Natural history, duplex characteristics and histopathologic correlation of arterial injuries in a canine model. *J Vasc Surg* 1992;16:867–876.

Parmley L, Mattingly T, Manion T. Nonpenetrating traumatic injury of the aorta. *Circulation* 1958;17:1086–1101.

Pate J, Gavant M, Weiman D, Fabian T. Traumatic rupture of the aortic isthmus: Program of selective management. *World J Surg* 1999;23:59–63.

Rasmusen TE, Clouse WD, Jenkins DH, Peck MA, Eliason JL, Smith DL. The use of temporary vascular shunts as a damage control adjunct in the management of wartime vascular injury. *J Trauma* 2006;61:8–15.

Rich NM. Principles and indications for primary venous repair. *Surgery* 1982;91:492.

Rich NM. Surgeons response to battlefield vascular trauma. *Am J Surg* 1993;166:91–96.

Rich NM, Hobson RW, Collins GJ, Andersen CA. The effect of acute popliteal venous interruption. *Ann Surg* 1976;183:365.

Risgaard O, Sugrue M, D'Amours S et al. Blunt cerebrovascular injury: An evaluation from a major trauma centre. *ANZ J Surg* 2007;77:686–689.

Rogers FB, Baker EF, Osler TM, Shackford SR, Wald SL, Vieco P. Computed tomographic angiography as a screening modality for blunt cervical arterial injuries: Preliminary results. *J Trauma* 1999;46:380–385.

Rosengart M, Smith DR, Melton SM, May AK, Rue LW 3rd. Prognostic factors in patients with inferior vena cava injuries. *Am Surg* 1999;65:849–856.

Schwartz MR, Weaver FA, Bauer M, Siegel A, Yellin AE. Refining the indications for arteriography in penetrating extremity trauma: A prospective analysis. *J Vasc Surg* 1993;17:116.

Shalhub S, Starnes BW, Tran NT et al. Blunt abdominal aortic injury. *J Vasc Surg* 2012;55:1277–1285.

Shapiro MB, Jenkins DH, Schwab CW, Rotondo MF. Damage control: Collective review. *J Trauma* 2000;49:969–978.

Stain SC, Yellin AE, Weaver FA, Pentecost MJ. Selective management of nonocclusive arterial injuries. *Arch Surg* 1989;124:1136–1141.

Stewart MK, Stone HH. Injuries of the inferior vena cava. *Am Surg* 1986;51:9–13.

Stone HH, Fabian TC, Turkleson ML. Wounds of the portal venous system. *World J Surg* 1982;6:335–341.

Subramanian A, Vercruysse G, Dente C, Wyrzykowski A, King E, Feliciano DV. A decades experience with temporary intravascular shunts at a civilian level I trauma center. *J Trauma* 2008;65:316–326.

Taller J, Kamder JP, Greene JA et al. Temporary vascular shunts as initial treatment of proximal extremity vascular injuries during combat operations: The new standard of care at echelon II facilities? *J Trauma* 2008;65:595–603.

Williams JS, Graff JA, Uku JM, Steinig JP. Aortic injury in vehicular trauma. *Ann Thorac Surg* 1994;57:726–730.

Zorilla P, Marin A, Gomez LA, Salido JA. Shoelace technique for gradual closure of fasciotomy wounds. *J Trauma* 2005;59:1515–1517.

6 Fasciotomy of the Extremities

Mark W. Bowyer

All surgeons involved in the care of traumatic injuries must have a working understanding of compartment syndrome (CS) of the extremities and be prepared to perform a fasciotomy as required. *CS is a limb-threatening and potentially life-threatening condition.* Long bone fractures and vascular injuries are the most frequent antecedent events, but other injuries such as burns, crush injury, bleeding into enclosed cavity spaces, external compression of a limb, thrombotic or embolic events, envenomation, allergy, intravenous infiltration, muscle overuse, nephritic syndrome and intramuscular injection have all been described as the underlying aetiology.

Pathophysiology

CS may occur wherever an anatomical compartment exists: Hand, forearm, upper arm, abdomen, buttock and the entire lower extremity (thigh & calf). The anatomical leg (calf) is the area most commonly affected, accounting for 68% in one large series, followed by the forearm (14%) and thigh (9%). These groups of muscles and their associated nerves and vessels are surrounded by thick, inelastic fascial layers that define the compartment boundaries, which are of relatively fixed volume.

As the pressure within a compartment rises (e.g. blood, fluid, oedema, external compression), the tissue perfusion inversely decreases leading to impaired cellular metabolism and cell death. If the pressure is not released in a timely fashion (historically reported as 4–6 hours, but may be as little as 1 hour in the shocked, polytrauma patient), irreversible tissue damage will occur. You must keep in mind that polytrauma patients with hypotension can sustain irreversible tissue injury at lower compartment pressures compared with patients with a normal blood pressure or MAP (mean arterial pressure), and thus, a high index of suspicion should be maintained in this group of patients.

Diagnosis

The diagnosis of compartment syndrome is a **clinical** one. The classically described five P's – *pain*, pallor, paresthesia, paralysis and pulselessness – are pathognomonic of compartment syndrome. However, *these are usually late signs and extensive, irreversible injury may already have taken place by the time they manifest.* The most important symptom is *pain greater than expected due to the injury alone.* But this may not be appreciated in the distracted, polytrauma or head injured patient. Remember that the loss of a distal pulse is a very late finding, and conversely the presence of pulses does not rule out CS, nor does the presence of open wounds exclude it either. In fact, more complex open fractures are associated with a higher prevalence of CS. Tissue pressure (compartment pressure) measurements have a limited role in diagnosis and are prone to both false positive and false negative error. The diagnosis is always clinical, and for any patient manifesting with signs and symptoms as described earlier or if a high index of suspicion is present (based on injury pattern and ischaemic time) expeditious compartment release is mandated. In patients with polytrauma CS, a diagnosis of exclusion and a low threshold for performing fasciotomy (especially after vascular injury) should be maintained. The safest approach is to *err* on the side of early and aggressive intervention and if one thinks about potentially doing a fasciotomy then it should be done, as this will also serve as prophylaxis even if not definitively therapeutic.

Treatment

The definitive treatment for compartment syndrome is *early and aggressive fasciotomy.* In patients with vascular injury who require fasciotomy in conjunction with a vascular repair, it is sometimes preferable to perform the fasciotomy *before* performing the repair. The rationale for this is that the ischaemic compartment is likely to be already tight and thus will create inflow resistance to the vascular repair, making it susceptible to early thrombosis. In addition, repairs may be time-consuming, rendering further muscle ischaemia if not released early. In reality, modern practice would likely mandate rapid shunting of the vessel (and vein if injured concomitantly) followed by fasciotomy, followed by reassessment and definitive vessel repair (including vein if injured) as appropriate (i.e. if damage control is deemed unnecessary).

Leg compartment syndrome and fasciotomy

Anatomy

The leg (calf) is the most common site for CS requiring fasciotomy. There are four major tissue compartments bounded by investing muscle fascia (**Figure 6.1**):

1. Anterior compartment
2. Lateral compartment
3. Superficial posterior compartment
4. Deep posterior compartment

There are important anatomical arrangements within each compartment with unique structures and understanding these is key to performing a formal, proper and complete

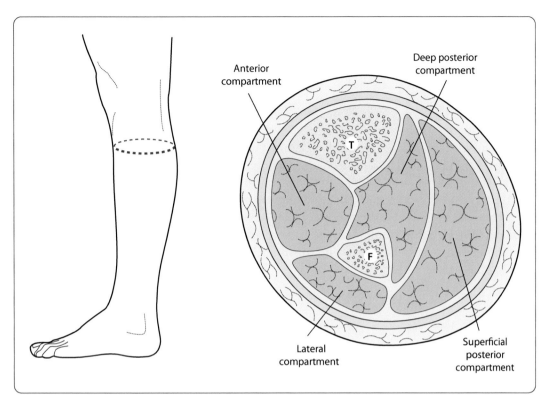

Figure 6.1 Cross-sectional anatomy of the mid-portion of the left lower leg depicting the four compartments that must be released when performing a lower leg fasciotomy. Statistically, the compartment most commonly missed is the anterior and deep posterior compartments. T = tibia, F = fibula.

four-compartment fasciotomy. It is not necessary to remember the names of all the muscles in each compartment, but it is useful to remember certain important details:

- The anterior compartment contains the anterior tibial artery and vein and the common peroneal nerve (recently renamed the common fibular nerve) (i.e. one artery and one nerve)
- The lateral compartment contains the superficial peroneal nerve (recently renamed the superior fibular nerve) which must not be injured (i.e. one nerve)
- The superficial posterior compartment contains the soleus and gastrocnemius muscles
- The deep posterior compartment contains the posterior tibial and peroneal vessels and the tibial nerve (i.e. two arteries and one nerve)

Technique

When managing the injured extremity, there is absolutely no role for being conservative or cosmetic and the oft-described 'single incision four-compartment fasciotomy' or 'closed-incision fasciotomy' are only mentioned as an act of condemnation. Attempts to make cosmetic incisions should also be condemned and the mantra should be 'bigger is better'. Compartment syndrome of the lower extremity after trauma dictates a *two-incision four-compartment fasciotomy* with *generous* skin openings.

The most commonly missed compartments during surgical decompression are the **anterior** and the **deep posterior**, and key to preventing this is correct placement of the skin incisions, especially as many of these extremities are already grossly swollen or deformed. Marking the key landmarks with a skin marker will aid in planning the incisions.

Lateral incision

The anterior tibial spine serves as a reliable midpoint between the incisions, and the lateral malleolus and fibular head are used to identify the course of the fibula on the lateral aspect (**Figure 6.2**). The lateral incision is made just anterior (~1 finger breadth above) to the line of the fibula, or *a finger in front of the fibula*. It is important to stay anterior to the fibula as this minimises the chance of damaging the superficial peroneal (superior fibular) nerve and helps to correctly identify the intermuscular septum between the anterior and lateral compartments. Some trauma surgeons advocate placing the lateral incision *midway* between the anterior tibial spine and the fibula for these very reasons and this is also an acceptable approach.

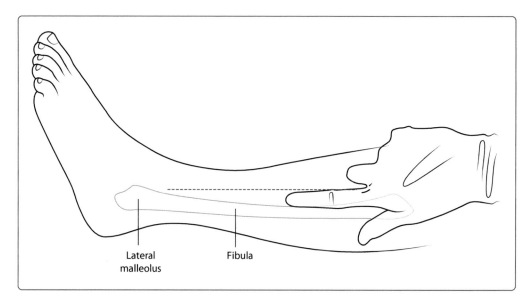

Lateral
malleolus

Fibula

Figure 6.2 The fibular head and lateral malleolus are used as reference points to mark the edge of the fibula and the lateral incision (dotted line) is made one finger in front of this (a finger in front of the fibula). The tibial spine serves as a midpoint reference between the two skin incisions. Alternatively, this lateral incision may also be made *midway* between the anterior spine of the tibia and the fibula.

Medial incision

The medial incision is made 1 thumb breadth below the palpable medial edge of the tibia (medial tibial border), or *a thumb below the tibia* (**Figure 6.3**). The extent of the skin incision should be to a point approximately 3 finger breadths below the tibial tuberosity and above the malleolus on either side.

It is very important to mark the incisions on both sides prior to opening them, as the landmarks of the swollen extremity will become rapidly distorted once the incision is made.

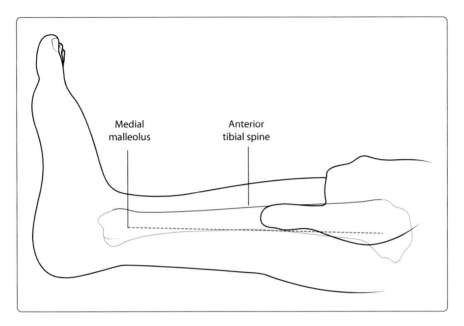

Figure 6.3 The medial incision (dotted line) is made 1 thumb breadth below the palpable medial edge of the tibia (solid line) (a thumb behind the tibia).

The lateral incision of the lower leg

As described, the lateral incision (**Figure 6.2**) is made *one finger in front if the fibula* and in general the incision runs from about 3 finger breadths below the head of the fibula to 3 finger breadths above the lateral malleolus. The exact length of the skin incision will depend on the clinical setting. Care is taken to make sure that it is long enough so that the skin does not serve as a constricting band, even if the fascia is adequately opened. The skin and subcutaneous tissue are incised to expose the fascia (white) encasing the lateral and anterior compartments. Care should be taken to avoid the respective peroneal (fibular) nerve when making the incision.

A gentle skin flap is raised using electrocautery and the intermuscular septum is identified. This divides the anterior from the lateral compartment. In the swollen or injured extremity, it may be difficult to identify, but identification is aided by following the perforating vessels down to it (**Figure 6.4a**). Classically the fascia of the lower leg is opened using an *H*-shaped incision. The crosspiece of the *H* using a scalpel which will expose both compartments and the septum must cross the intermuscular septum. The legs of the *H* are made with a curved scissors using just the tips which are turned away from the septum to avoid injury to the peroneal (fibular) nerve (**Figures 6.4b** and **6.5**). The fascia is opened by pushing the partially opened scissor tips in both directions (cephalad and caudad) on either side of the septum opening the fascia from the head of the fibula down to the lateral malleolus. Inspection of the septum and identification of the common peroneal (fibular) nerve and/or the anterior tibial vessels confirms entry into the anterior compartment. The skin incision should be closely inspected and extended as needed to ensure that the ends do not serve as a point of further constriction. Ensure good haemostasis along the skin edges and any branches from the superficial veins.

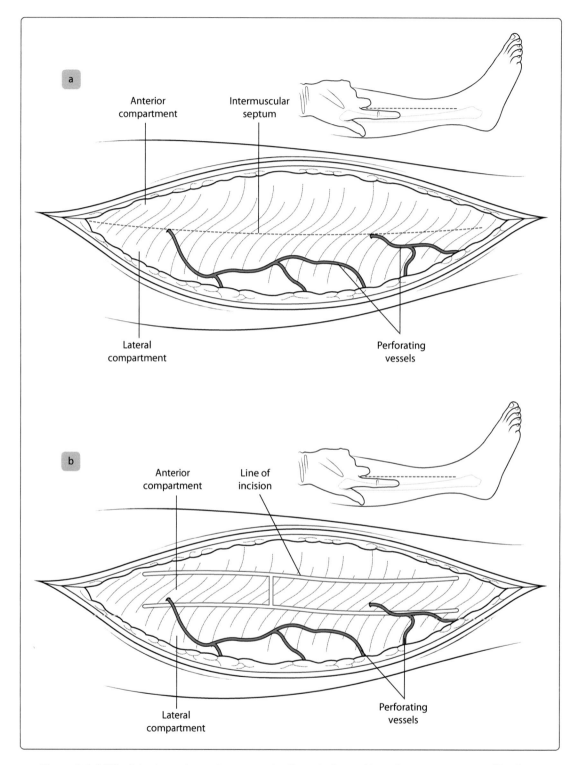

Figure 6.4 (a) The intermuscular septum separates the anterior and lateral compartments and is where the perforating vessels exit. (b) The fascia overlying the anterior and lateral compartments is opened in an *H*-shaped fashion.

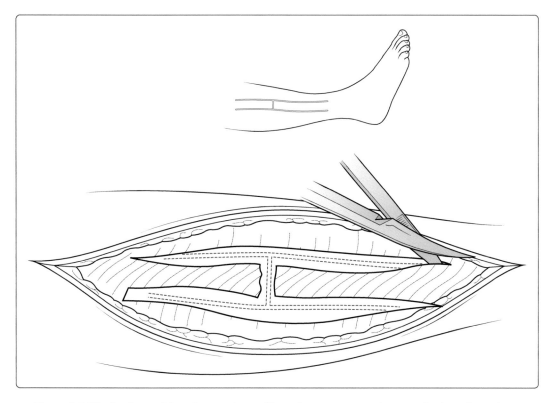

Figure 6.5 The fascia overlying the anterior and lateral compartments is opened using scissors in an *H*-shaped fashion with the scissor tips turned away from the septum.

The medial incision of the lower leg

As described, the medial incision (**Figure 6.3**) is made 1 finger breadth below the palpable medial edge of the tibia (*one thumb behind the tibia*). When making this incision, it is important to identify and preferably preserve the greater saphenous vein and ligate any tributaries to it. In most individuals, the fascia next encountered directly overlies the superficial posterior compartment (soleus and gastrocnemius muscle) and exposure is further enhanced by raising gentle overlying skin flaps. The fascia is opened from the tibial tuberosity to the medial malleolus, effectively decompressing the superficial compartment (**Figure 6.6**). The gatekeeper to entering the deep posterior compartment is the soleus muscle, as it attaches medially to the under surface of the posterior tibia. The soleus muscle attaches to the medial edge of the tibia, and dissecting these fibres completely free from and exposing the underside of the tibia (relatively avascular plane if entered correctly) ensures entry into the deep posterior compartment (**Figure 6.7**). Identification of the posterior tibial neurovascular bundle confirms that the correct compartment has been entered. The muscle in each compartment should be assessed for viability. *Viable muscle is pink, contracts when stimulated and bleeds when cut.* Dead muscle should be debrided back to healthy viable tissue. Ensure good haemostasis along the skin edges and any branches from the superficial veins. The skin incision is left open and either covered with gauze or a vacuum-assisted wound closure device, which have been shown in recent studies to speed up and improve the chances for definitive closure of these wounds.

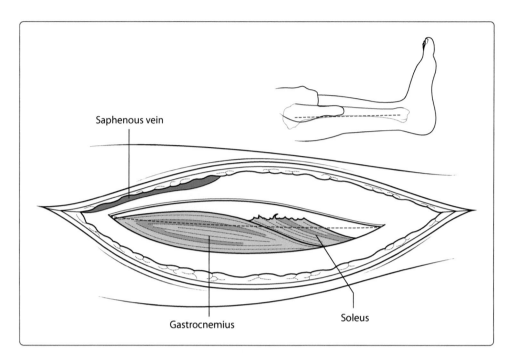

Figure 6.6 The medial incision is placed such that the great saphenous vein can be identified and preserved, and the fascia is opened to expose the soleus and gastrocnemius muscles in the superficial posterior compartment.

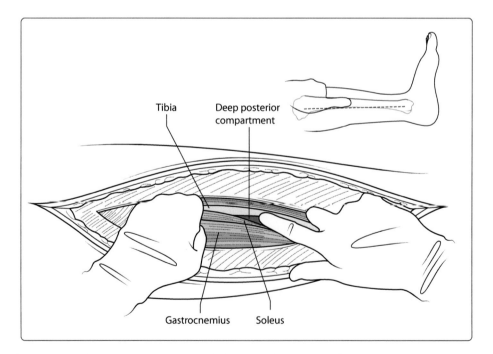

Figure 6.7 The soleus muscle is dissected off of the posterior border of the tibia allowing entry into the deep posterior compartment.

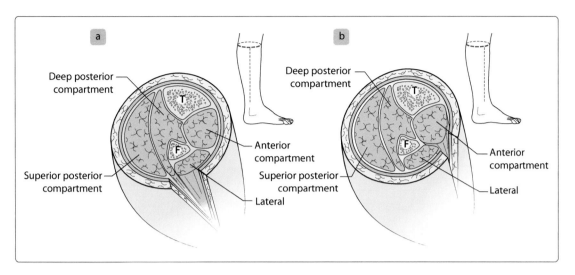

Figure 6.8 (a) When the lateral incision is made too far posterior, the septum between the lateral and superficial posterior compartments may be mistaken for that between the anterior and lateral leading to the anterior compartment not being opened. (b) When the lateral incision is made one finger in front of the fibula, the septum between the anterior and lateral compartments is more readily identified allowing for adequate decompression of both the anterior and lateral compartments.

Pitfalls

The biggest pitfall is failure to identify and adequately open all four compartments. Statistically, the anterior compartment is most commonly missed, typically because the skin incision is made too far posteriorly, either directly over or behind the fibula, thereby failing to recognise and enter the anterior compartment completely or at all. When the incision is made in this manner the septum between the lateral and the superficial compartment may be directly below the incision and is erroneously identified as the septum between the anterior and lateral compartments (**Figure 6.8a**). When the lateral incision is made *one finger in front of the fibula*, the intramuscular septum between the anterior and lateral compartments is found directly below the incision making successful decompression more likely (**Figure 6.8b**).

The deep posterior compartment can also be missed, and a thorough understanding of the anatomy is key to ensuring that this does not happen. Many surgeons do not appreciate that the fibres of the muscle must be dissected free from off the under surface of the tibia to allow adequate entry into the deep compartment and it is not a fascial incision *per se* at this stage. Another pitfall to successful opening of the deep posterior compartment is inadvertent entry into the plane between the gastrocnemius and soleus muscle (rather than behind the bony tibia), thereby giving the impression to the less experienced surgeon that the compartment has been successfully released (**Figure 6.9a**). *Proper decompression of the deep posterior compartment requires that the soleus fibres are separated from their attachment on the underside of the tibia* (**Figures 6.7 and 6.9b**).

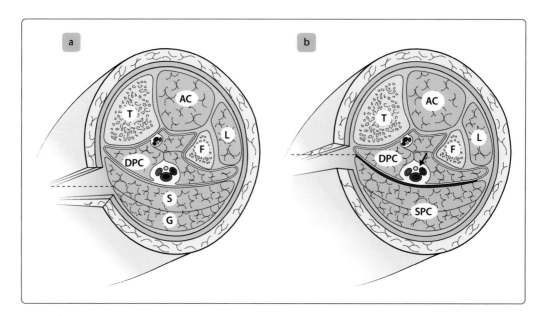

Figure 6.9 (a) A potential pitfall when performing the medial incision is to develop a plane inadvertently between the gastrocnemius (G) and soleus (S) muscles and believing that this represents the plane between the superficial (SPC) and deep posterior (DPC) compartment. (b) Entry into and release of the deep posterior compartment requires separating both the gastrocnemius and soleus from the underside of the tibia. Identification of the neurovascular bundle (arrow) confirms that the deep posterior compartment has been entered. T = tibia, F = fibula.

Compartment syndrome of the thigh

Compartment syndrome is uncommon in the thigh because of the large volume required to increase the interstitial pressure. In addition, the compartments of the thigh blend anatomically with the hip allowing for extravasation of blood or fluid outside the compartment. Major risk factors for thigh compartment syndrome include; femoral fractures, vascular injury, severe blunt trauma/crush or blast injury, direct trauma to the muscle and external compression of the thigh. The thigh contains three compartments: anterior, posterior and medial. If decompression is required, start with a lateral incision as this enables decompression of both the anterior and posterior compartments (**Figure 6.10**). Typically, only the lateral incision is required, though on occasion with a severely swollen extremity, a medial incision may also be required (**Figure 6.10**).

The single lateral incision is made one finger breadth above the tensor fascia lata (condensed fascia running from the greater tuberosity of the hip to the lateral aspect of the knee and is palpated as a tense, firm band of tissue). A skin flap is raised above and below this incision, exposing the fascia investing the anterior and posterior compartments respectively. Two separate longitudinal incisions are made in each of these compartments and a *H* incision created, crossing the tense fascial band of the tensor fascia lata to ensure both compartments have been entered. This is typically adequate to decompress the entire thigh.

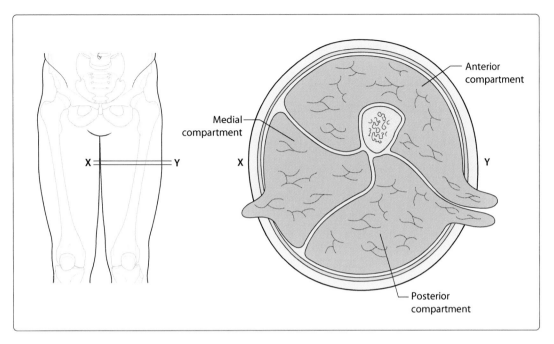

Figure 6.10 The thigh has three compartments: anterior, posterior and medial. The anterior and posterior compartments of the thigh are decompressed through a single lateral incision. On occasion, the medial compartment will need decompression through a separate medial incision.

Compartment syndrome of the forearm and hand

Compartment syndrome of the hand and forearm are much less common compared with the lower extremity, but are vital to recognise and treat, as a missed upper limb CS may be a lot more disabling than a lower limb one, especially if the dominant arm is involved (limb loss, chronic limb ischaemia, neurological compromise, muscle contracture and chronic painful neuritis). Although unusual, upper limb CS may occur following supracondylar fracture of the humerus, vascular injury, crush or blast injury and burns. CS of the hand may occur after trauma but is more commonly associated with infiltration of intravenous fluids. As there are no large sensory nerves in the hand compartments, physical findings do not typically include sensory abnormalities, and the pressure threshold for release is much lower compared with the lower limb (15–20 mm Hg).

The literature is replete with numerous descriptions of the various ways to perform the skin incisions to open the compartments of the forearm. The most commonly used and described technique is a curvilinear incision along the volar (flexor) surface (to release the anterior or volar compartments), which is extended to the hand to release the carpal tunnel (**Figure 6.11**). This is the most important compartment as it contains the flexors for normal hand function. The incision is typically started at the medial aspect of the distal humerus (i.e. above the elbow joint and where the inflow vessels to the forearm [brachial artery] may be controlled if required) and extended across the antecubital fossa as a gentle curvilinear incision (to avoid a skin contracture across the joint). The incision then traverses the forearm volar surface at least once in a curvilinear fashion (to ensure the compartment

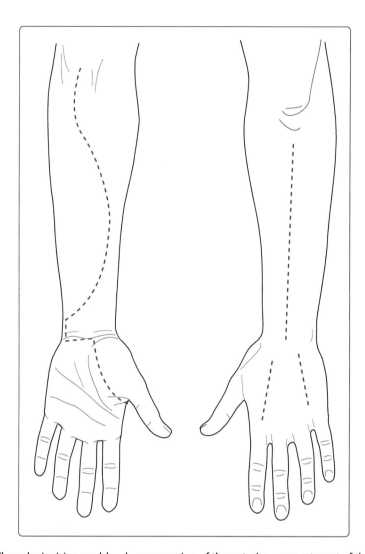

Figure 6.11 The volar incision enables decompression of the anterior compartment of the forearm and is carried down onto the hand to release the carpal tunnel. The incision on the volar aspect must cross the width of the forearm at least once (to avoid a contracture afterwards), but this is unnecessary on the dorsum. The dorsal incision allows for decompression of the posterior compartment and the two dorsal hand incisions enable release of the intraosseous compartments.

is adequately decompressed and to avoid a skin contracture across the flexor muscles) and then across the flexor retinaculum of the wrist and into the palmer fascia for 1–2 cm (often following the curve of the thenar eminence). The fascia encountered below the skin incision is much thinner in comparison to the lower limb (except the palmer fascia which is even thicker). The fascia is opened along the same incision line as the skin incision. In addition, the flexor retinaculum must be opened (take care not to injure the median nerve here) and the palmer fascia divided for 1–2 cm.

The posterior compartment of the forearm is released through a linear (or slightly semi-lunar) dorsal incision and does not require the same extensive format as the volar aspect. Two additional incisions on the dorsum of the hand to release the hand compartment may also be used (**Figure 6.11**). The rationale for the placement of these incisions is a better cosmetic and functional result as well as maintenance of an adequate blood supply to the skin between the two skin flaps. Additionally, this incision allows for a vascularised skin flap to cover and protect the median nerve and the flexor tendons at the wrist.

Aftercare and complications

If necrotic muscle is present, it should be debrided at the time of original fasciotomy, which, as described earlier, will create large wounds that must be covered. The open wounds should be covered with non-adherent dressing or moist gauze. If you have access to a vacuum-assisted wound closure device, application to the wound will help to protect the tissue and may speed time to wound closure. The wounds should be re-evaluated 24–48 hours after the initial fasciotomy with further debridement as indicated. After the acute process subsides, delayed primary closure or split-thickness skin grafting may be performed. Patients with open fasciotomy wounds are at risk for infection, and incomplete or delayed fasciotomies can lead to permanent nerve damage, loss of limb, multisystem organ failure, rhabdomyolysis and death. Early recognition and aggressive fasciotomy will help to minimise these adverse outcomes.

Important points

1. Compartment syndrome must be suspected in all polytrauma patients especially if hypotensive.
2. Compartment syndrome is a clinical diagnosis. There is a very limited role for measuring compartment pressures.
3. The earliest and most important symptom of compartment syndrome is pain greater than expected due to the injury alone.
4. The presence of pulses and normal capillary refill does not exclude compartment syndrome.
5. If you wait for the five P's to make a diagnosis of compartment syndrome, your patient will be left with the sixth P – a peg leg.
6. The presence of an open fracture does not exclude compartment syndrome and in fact may make it more likely.
7. The lower leg is the most common site of compartment syndrome followed by the forearm and thigh.
8. Fasciotomies performed for trauma must include generous skin incisions and complete release of the fascia. The skin can act as a constricting band even if the fascia is fully opened.
9. Lower extremity four-compartment fasciotomy must be done through two skin incisions. There is no role for the one skin incision fasciotomy in the lower leg.
10. The lateral incision is made a finger in front of the fibula.
11. The medial incision is made a thumb below the tibia.
12. A cosmetic incision for compartment syndrome equals an improper fasciotomy.
13. In the swollen lower leg, the lateral intermuscular septum can be difficult to find and the perforating vessels will help you locate it.
14. Taking the time to mark all the landmarks and proposed incisions prior to cutting will improve your chances of successful fasciotomy.

15. The anterior and deep posterior compartments of the lower extremity are the most commonly missed compartments. Identifying the respective neurovascular structures in each compartment confirms you have entered them.

16. Necrotic muscle does not contract when electrocautery is applied. It must be debrided at the time of the initial fasciotomy.

17. Compartment syndrome of the foot and hand are infrequent, and best outcomes are obtained in conjunction with subspecialty input.

Additional reading

Bowyer MW. Lower extremity fasciotomy: Indications and technique. *Curr Trauma Rep* 2015;1:35–44

Bowyer MW. Compartment syndrome and lower extremity fasciotomy. In Gahtan V, Costanza M, eds. *Essentials of Vascular Surgery for the General Surgeon*. Philadelphia: Springer, 2015:55–71.

Branco BC, Inaba K, Barmparas G et al. Incidence and predictors for the need for fasciotomy after extremity trauma: A 10-year review in a mature level I trauma centre. *Injury* 2011;42:1157–1163.

Dente CJ, Feliciano DV, Rozycki GS et al. A review of upper extremity fasciotomies in a level 1 trauma center. *Am Surg* 2004;70:1088–1093.

Feliciano DV, Cruse PA, Spjut-Patrinely V. Fasciotomy after trauma to the extremities. *Am J Surg* 1988;156:533–536.

Garner MR, Taylor SA, Gausden E, Lyden JP. Compartment syndrome: Diagnosis, management, and unique concerns in the twenty-first century. *HSS J* 2014;10:143–152.

Kalyani BS, Fisher BE, Roberts CS, Giannoudis PV. Compartment syndrome of the forearm: A systematic review. *J Hand Surg Am* 2011;36:535–543.

Ojike N, Roberts C, Giannoudis P. Compartment syndrome of the thigh: A systematic review. *Injury* 2010;41:133–136.

Ritenour AE, Dorlac WC, Fang R et al. Complications after fasciotomy revision and delayed compartment release in combat patients. *J Trauma* 2008;64(2 Suppl):S153–S162.

Schwartz JT, Brumback RJ, Lakatos R et al. Acute compartment syndrome of the thigh. A spectrum of injury. *J Bone Joint Surg Am* 1989;71:392–400.

Shadgan B, Menon M, O'Brien PJ, Reid WD. Diagnostic techniques in acute compartment syndrome of the leg. *J Orthop Trauma* 2008;22:581–587.

Smith J, Bowyer MW. Fasciotomy of the forearm and hand. In Demeitriades D, Inaba K, Velmahos G, eds. *Atlas of Surgical Techniques in Trauma*. Cambridge: Cambridge University Press, 2015:288–293.

Zannis J, Angobaldo J, Marks M et al. Comparison of fasciotomy wound closures using traditional dressing changes and vacuum-assisted closure device. *Ann Plast Surg* 2009;62:407–409.

7

Damage Control for Severe Pelvic Haemorrhage in Trauma

John H. Armstrong

Objectives

1. Define sources of haemorrhage in patients sustaining high-energy pelvic fractures
2. Discuss options for temporary and definitive control of exsanguinating pelvic haemorrhage
3. Describe the steps necessary to perform extraperitoneal pelvic packing

Up to 13% of patients sustaining blunt pelvic fractures will present in shock. These patients with high-energy pelvic fractures have multiple, coincident sources of potential haemorrhage beyond the pelvis, including the chest and abdomen, with a 30% mortality rate. Attribution of pelvic haemorrhage as the cause of death is confounded by multiple sources of haemorrhage, as well as accompanying traumatic brain injury (TBI) and subsequent multi-system organ failure from high-energy trauma. To save these lives, a comprehensive approach is required to;

1. Identify the pelvis as a primary or contributing source of exsanguinating haemorrhage
2. Intervene quickly to stop the bleeding

Pelvic anatomy and haemorrhage

The bony pelvis includes the three paired bones of the pubis, ilium and ischium, and a single sacrum posteriorly; together, they form an antero-inferior tilted bony cavity (**Figure 7.1**). The bones are connected anteriorly by the ligamentous public symphysis and

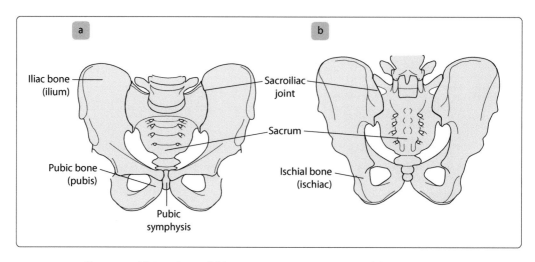

Figure 7.1 (a) Anterior and (b) posterior anatomic images of the bony pelvis.

posteriorly by the sacroiliac joints and multiple ligaments (sacrospinous, sacrotuberous and iliolumbar). When the pubic symphysis and sacroiliac ligaments are disrupted, the volume of the pelvic basin increases and has greater capacity for collecting haemorrhage in the pelvic retroperitoneal space. The pubis has two rami, superior and inferior, that join the ischium to form the obturator foramina. The pelvic cavity not only contains organs of the urogenital and lower gastrointestinal tracts, but also the transiting lower extremity neurovasculature and a dense concentration of blood vessels for the pelvic viscera and muscles. A rich venous plexus, in particular, is tethered to the pelvic walls, posterior and adherent to named arteries, which are vulnerable to laceration with pelvic fractures. Two branches of the internal iliac artery are also at particular risk of laceration with severe pelvic fractures, namely, the superior gluteal and internal pudendal arteries. The fractured surfaces of the pelvic bones themselves can bleed as well. Thus, there are three primary sources of pelvic bleeding after pelvic fracture:

1. Venous plexus (80% of all pelvic bleeding)
2. Arterial branches (10%–15% of open-book pelvic fractures and 75% of haemodynamically unstable pelvic fractures)
3. Cancellous bony ends of fractures

The pelvis is like a hard pretzel in that one cannot break a pretzel in one place alone: it always breaks in at least two places. Structures (including vasculature) in proximity to the fractures can be injured, especially the pelvic veins. The pelvic cavity pressure is lower than venous and arterial pressures and has a large potential retroperitoneal space for haemorrhage and clot to fill. The pelvic organs are readily compressed or displaced upwards into the abdomen, enabling an even larger potential space to fill with blood. It is rare for the peritoneum overlying the clot and blood to rupture freely into the peritoneum; instead the pelvic peritoneum continues to auto-dissect away from the bony pelvis in all directions (posteriorly, laterally and anteriorly), creating more space for further haemorrhage. Exsanguinating pelvic haemorrhage is typically associated with arterial bleeding in combination with venous haemorrhage.

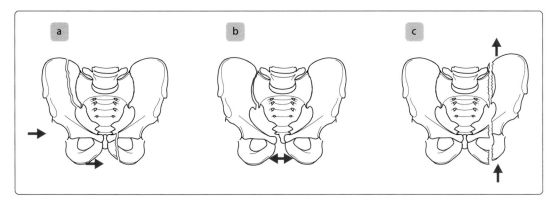

Figure 7.2 Severe pelvic fractures. (a) Lateral compression fracture. (b) Anterior-posterior compression (open book) fracture. (c) Vertical shear fracture.

The pelvic bones and ligaments are sturdy structures and therefore require a significantly large amount of energy to break (e.g. high energy motor vehicle collision [MVC], falls >2 M, and pedestrian versus motor vehicle). There are three broad patterns of severe pelvic fracture (**Figure 7.2**):

1. Lateral compression
2. Anterior-posterior (A-P) compression ('open book')
3. Vertical shear

In high-speed MVCs, it is not unusual to see a combination of these pelvic injury patterns. However, if an A-P compression injury is present, this will open the pelvic ring, thereby increasing the potential space for blood to collect in the pelvic retroperitoneum, aggravating haemorrhage and the potential for exsanguination.

Damage control for pelvic haemorrhage

As previously emphasised, recognition of exsanguinating haemorrhage in the injured patient is the first critical step in management. The mechanism of injury will define the amount and vector of energy that has caused the injury and therefore the potential for bleeding. Thus, the mechanism component of ATMIST (i.e. Age-Time of Injury-Mechanism-Injuries-(Vital) Signs-Treatment) is particularly salient in the evaluation (i.e. the mechanism predicts the likelihood of significant pelvic trauma, the likely constellation of injuries and potential for major haemorrhage). CAB (i.e. Circulation-Airway-Breathing) assessment demonstrates present or emerging shock, and the massive transfusion protocol should be initiated.

A rapid diagnosis of significant pelvic fracture (and thus a potential source of haemorrhage) begins with the clinical examination. Palpation along the pelvic margins may elicit tenderness in the lucid patient. Perineal bruising, blood at the urethral meatus, and a high-riding prostate (absent prostate on digital rectal exam) may be additional clues of pelvic fracture, but in themselves are not reliable. Only a single, gentle attempt to assess for A-P stability with simultaneous palmar pressure on the anterior superior iliac spines should be performed. Aggressive pelvic manipulation, such as 'springing the pelvis' or 'open-booking the pelvis,' have the potential to aggravate bleeding and must not be done.

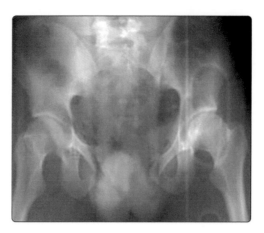

Figure 7.3 Anterior-posterior pelvic plain radiograph, demonstrating an anterior-posterior compression 'open book' pelvic fracture. (Image courtesy of Stephen L. Barnes, MD, FACS).

A rapid anterior-posterior plain radiograph of the pelvis gives a snapshot of the fracture patterns described earlier (**Figure 7.3**). A FAST (Focussed Assessment with Sonography for Trauma) scan may also demonstrate free fluid (i.e. blood) in the peritoneal cavity, but is not reliable to rule out pelvic bleeding if negative because pelvic bleeding from fractures is retroperitoneal. In the exsanguinating patient, there is no place for CT scan evaluation.

Once an unstable or potentially unstable pelvis has been recognised, external pelvic compression with a commercial pelvic binder or tight sheet should be rapidly applied. The binder or sheet must be centred on the greater trochanters of the femurs. The reduction in pelvic volume following the application of the binder provides initial haemorrhage control by reducing pelvic volume while other sources of bleeding are considered. The patient's response to resuscitation with the massive transfusion protocol also guides further assessment for haemorrhage sources. If the patient's haemodynamics improve and are well enough for transport and radiology, a CT scan of the chest-abdomen–pelvis may be considered, with the understanding that the patient must be monitored by the trauma team during transport and radiology.

If the patient remains haemodynamically unstable and uncontrolled pelvic haemorrhage remains a likely source, extraperitoneal pelvic packing should be performed: **packs are placed deliberately within the pelvic extraperitoneal space to achieve direct compression and tamponade low-pressure venous bleeding**. This can be performed in the prepared emergency department or in theatre, either with or without laparotomy.

For the majority of patients presenting with major haemorrhage and a significant pelvic fracture, 90% will have associated injuries, 50% will have a compelling source of bleeding outside of the pelvis and 30% will have intra-abdominal haemorrhage. Therefore, if pelvic packing is required, then there is a very high chance that a laparotomy is also required for injuries within the abdomen. Extraperitoneal pelvic packing *via* a laparotomy is more commonly performed than pelvis-only pelvic packing (without laparotomy) when damage control surgery is indicated.

Still, there are occasions where pelvis-only extraperitoneal pelvic packing may suffice (e.g. isolated pelvic-only bleeding only is confirmed on follow-up CT). Pelvic packing should not interfere with laparotomy, and laparotomy should not be a deterrent to pelvic packing—the key is to keep the anterior pelvic peritoneum intact.

Technique of pelvis-only extraperitoneal pelvic packing

- Make a lower midline infra-umbilical incision (or occasionally a Pfannenstiel incision) through the skin, subcutaneous fat and linea alba (**Figure 7.4**).
- Enter the preperitoneal space by manually sweeping the peritoneal reflection in a superolateral direction along the inner table of the pelvis. Often in trauma, the pelvic haematoma will have done most of this dissection already, and the space is easier to identify and develop.

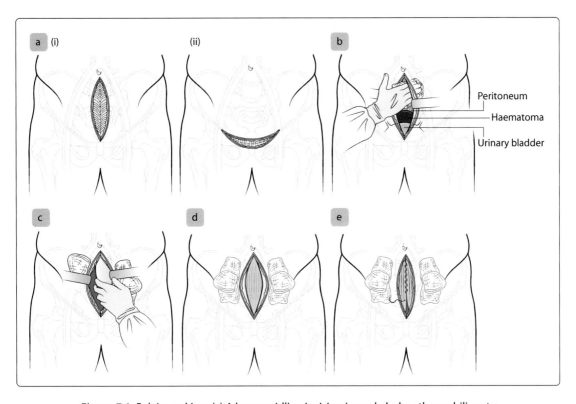

Figure 7.4 Pelvic packing. (a) A lower midline incision is made below the umbilicus to gain access to the true pelvis (i). Occasionally a transverse (Pfannenstiel) incision is used (ii). (b) The side walls of the opened abdominal wall are retracted widely open and the haematoma is appreciated (red), which may by now freely evacuate. (c) Rolled abdominal packs are placed deliberately and sequentially deep into the pelvic cavity, making sure to fill the space and compress against the bony ring. (d) Rolled abdominal packs are placed similarly on the opposite side, and the haemodynamic response is reassessed. (e) The fascia and/or skin may be closed to provide additional tamponade, though primary haemostasis occurs with the packing itself.

- Expose the space with assistant retraction of the anterior abdominal wall and manual compression of the peritoneum with the non-dominant hand. The large pelvic haematoma typically evacuates spontaneously, though clot may require manual removal.
- Place sequential rolled laparotomy sponges over the non-dominant hand and deep into the recesses of the pelvis, beginning at the sacro-iliac joint posteriorly and proceeding anteriorly. Typically three to five sponges are needed on each side.
- Take care not to violate the peritoneum, which will open up the intra-abdominal space and permit pelvic haemorrhage to decompress further into the larger peritoneal cavity. Small bowel can herniate through the peritoneal defect as well and obscure the surgical field for deliberate pelvic packing.
- Repeat the same process for pack placement on the opposite side. If effective packing has taken place, the superficial sponges on top should remain white.
- Close the skin rapidly with a running nylon suture to aid pelvic compression.
- Reassess patient response to resuscitation and pelvic packing haemostasis.

Technique of extraperitoneal pelvic packing *via* the abdomen

If a non-expanding pelvic haematoma (zone 3 retroperitoneal haematoma) is known or encountered during trauma laparotomy, it should be left intact because it has self-tamponaded. However, if the hematoma is expanding or pulsatile (indicative of arterial bleeding), then pelvic packing is mandatory and may be effectively performed through the same laparotomy incision. Note that zone 3 retroperitoneal haematomas from penetrating trauma must be explored (**Figure 7.5**).

- Identify the peritoneal reflection against the pelvic sidewall and, grasping the edge with surgical clips or Littlewood graspers, dissect the peritoneum away from the side wall.
- Ensure that the pelvic space is fully developed and evacuate the haematoma. Typically, the pelvic haematoma has done most of this dissection already, and the surgeon may only need to manually enlarge the space.
- Place rolled laparotomy sponges into the pelvic recesses sequentially and deliberately to compress any further bleeding. Typically, three to five sponges are needed on each side.
- Repeat the process on the opposite side.
- Consider damage control for injuries identified within the peritoneal cavity itself and transport the patient to the ITU (intensive therapy unit) for correction of pathophysiology.

Additional strategies

Once pelvic packing has been performed, the pelvic binder may be re-applied to provide additional tamponade of the bleeding by re-apposition of the open pelvic ring.

Angiography with selective embolisation of arterial bleeding branches should follow pelvic packing as an adjunct to achieve definitive haemorrhage control. Angiography is not appropriate for the exsanguinating patient. Non-selective embolisation (i.e. embolising the entire internal iliac close to origin) is an option for diffuse arterial bleeding, but if performed

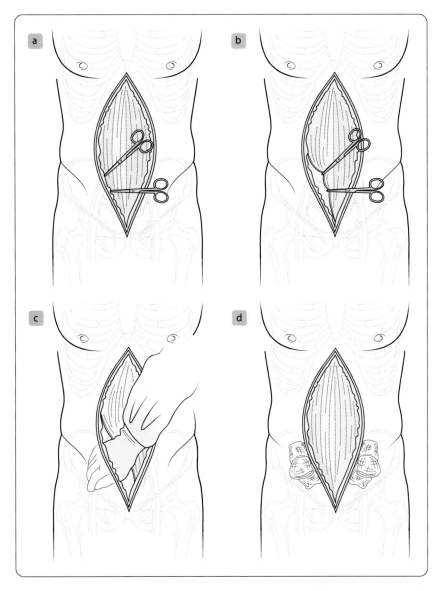

Figure 7.5 Pelvic packing *via* the abdomen (a). The edges of the pelvic peritoneal reflection are grasped with a surgical instrument to aid 'stripping' of the peritoneum from the side wall (b). Often a large and expanding haematoma has done this part of the dissection already (c). Once the space is opened, it may be developed further manually, before placing the rolled up surgical swabs deep inside the pelvis to create an artificial tamponade of the bleeding (d).

bilaterally, carries a risk of gluteal infarction. A member of the trauma team must monitor the patient during transport and throughout procedures in the interventional radiology suite.

Further surgical options for definitive haemorrhage control are rarely used because they necessitate opening the pelvic haematoma. Bilateral ligation of the internal iliac arteries is challenging in the setting of a pelvic haematoma that obscures the view of the internal iliac arteries. In addition, it does not control bleeding from the pelvic venous plexuses. Venous bleeding on the sacrum may be additionally controlled with sterile thumbtacks.

Damage control stage III

The use of some combination of pelvic binder, pelvic packing, and angioembolisation, coupled with the massive transfusion protocol, is very effective in achieving definitive control of pelvic haemorrhage from severe pelvic fractures. With bleeding controlled, the extraperitoneal pelvic packs should be removed following normalisation of haemodynamics, coagulation, temperature and pH (i.e. damage control surgery [DCS] stage II, Intensive Therapy Unit). This should be done in theatre within 48 hours, as after this time the risk of sepsis from packs increases exponentially.

External pelvic fracture fixation has a role in providing mechanical pelvic stability following control of exsanguinating haemorrhage but is not a damage control procedure. Such fixation takes at least an hour from request to completion. Pelvic fixation may be considered for pelvic mechanical stabilisation following haemorrhage control (i.e. DCS stage III).

Assessment for urethral, bladder, rectal, and vaginal injuries should be conducted after definitive haemorrhage control. If there is a rectal injury or an open pelvic fracture through the pelvic floor, a defunctioning colostomy may be performed during DCS stage III. The stoma in the open abdomen should be placed more cephalad and lateral to an elective stoma site to keep it well out of the surgical field.

Additional reading

Costantini TW, Coimbra R, Holcomb JB et al. Current management of hemorrhage from severe pelvic fractures: Results of an American Association for the Surgery of Trauma multi-institutional trial. *J Trauma Acute Care Surg* 2016;80(5):717–725.

Croce MA, Magnotti LJ, Savage SA, Wood GW II, Fabian TC. Emergent pelvic fixation in patients with exsanguinating pelvic fractures. *J Am Coll Surg* 2007;204:935–942.

Cullinane DC, Schiller HJ, Zielinski MD et al. Eastern Association for the surgery of trauma practice management guidelines for hemorrhage in pelvic fracture—Update and systematic review. *J Trauma* 2011;71:1850–1868.

Davis JW, Moore FA, McIntyre RC Jr, Cocanour CS, Moore EE, West MA. Western Trauma Association critical decisions in trauma: Management of pelvic fracture with hemodynamic instability. *J Trauma* 2008;65:1012–1015.

DuBose J, Inaba K, Barfmparas G et al. Bilateral internal iliac artery ligation as a damage control approach in massive retroperitoneal bleeding after pelvic fracture. *J Trauma* 2010;69:1507–1514.

Flint L, Cryer G. Pelvic fracture: The last 50 years. *J Trauma* 2010;69:483–88.

Jeske HC, Larndorder R, Krappinger D et al. Management of hemorrhage in severe pelvic injuries. *J Trauma* 2010;68:415–420.

Mauffrey C, Cueller DO II, Pieracci F et al. Strategies for the management of haemorrhage following pelvic fractures and associated trauma-induced coagulopathy. *Bone Joint J* 2014;96-B:1143–1154.

Miller PR, Moore PS, Mansell E, Meredith JW, Chang MC. External fixation or arteriogram in bleeding pelvic fracture: Initial therapy guided by markers of arterial hemorrhage. *J Trauma* 2003;54:437–443.

Totterman A, Madsen JE, Skaga NO, Roise O. Extraperitoneal pelvic packing: A salvage procedure to control massive traumatic pelvic hemorrhage. *J Trauma* 2007;62:843–852.

8

Trauma Laparotomy and Damage Control Laparotomy

David M. Nott

The goal of the standard trauma laparotomy in the patient with *relative* haemodynamic stability is *rapid access to the abdominal cavity* followed by immediate and rapid *control of the compelling source of bleeding*. Following this, a rapid but complete abdominal exploration is performed to define all injuries. The surgeon must then decide if this standard trauma laparotomy must now become a 'damage control' one, as determined by the patient's own physiology and response to surgery.

The goal of the damage control (abbreviated) laparotomy is to immediately treat severe haemorrhage and secondly contain contamination in those patients whose physiologic and metabolic condition is likely to deteriorate with continued, prolonged or extensive surgery. This decision may be taken pre-emptively before or at the outset of surgery (based on physiology and/or injury burden) or at any time after the standard trauma laparotomy has begun, should the patient's physiologic and metabolic state demand it. Instead of performing a full, complete and definitive operation, once gross haemorrhage and contamination control are achieved, this is immediately followed by abdominal packing, temporary abdominal closure and termination of further surgery (for now!).

Who needs damage control surgery?

The decision to perform the abbreviated form of the trauma laparotomy is determined by several factors, both anatomical and physiological. Anatomical factors include;

- Injury burden (multisystem trauma patient)
- Complex injuries (likely to fail at the index procedure such as complex duodenal/pancreatic injuries, need for prolonged vascular bypass)

- Other more compelling injuries in need of priority treatment (e.g. traumatic brain injury [TBI])
- Any injury that may require a relook procedure anyway (e.g. bowel of questionable viability)

Physiologic factors are determined by the metabolic state of end-organ tissue perfusion (i.e. the *trauma triad of death* as described in Chapter 1), such as;

- Acidosis (pH, lactate, BE)
- Temperature (hypothermia)
- Coagulopathy

For this group of patients, an immediate surgical procedure to rapidly save a life is indicated, as a prolonged operation will worsen physiological impairment, typically ending in catastrophic failure (i.e. death). Those patients who have lost a significant volume of blood if not treated expeditiously will quickly become (if not already depending on injury severity, magnitude of haemorrhage and time since injury) *coagulopathic, hypothermic* and *acidotic* – the *trauma triad of death*. Additional decisions to perform an abbreviated laparotomy may also include;

- The number of casualties in need of emergency surgery (i.e. mass casualty situation)
- Your own surgical skill set (i.e. do enough to save a life / limb, then wait for additional skills or transfer out as appropriate)

Although there is no absolute time cut-off for damage control surgery (DCS), we always aim to have all bleeding and contamination under control within 60 minutes and transfer to the intensive care unit (ICU) within 90 minutes. Some surgeons advocate that this is even too long in the truly exsanguinating patient.

Damage control laparotomy

Uncontrollable or sustained bleeding within the abdomen mandates immediate laparotomy. A rapid sequence of steps are followed in a methodical fashion to arrest haemorrhage, contain contamination and maintain end-organ perfusion and oxygenation so that any physiological deterioration is halted and allowed to recover. It is not justifiable to continue further surgery at this stage. After a period of physiological improvement in the ICU, where the hypothermia, acidosis and coagulopathy are reversed (which may take 24–72 hours), definitive anatomical re-look surgery is scheduled.

The venue

Surgery must take place in a warm (environmental temperature set at 30°C) operating theatre that is well equipped for 'all cavity' surgery with monitoring equipment, adequate lighting and access to blood and blood products. We do not advocate ever performing a laparotomy outside of the operating suite, including the emergency department, despite heroic claims to the contrary.

The surgical field must expose the patient from neck to knee (potentially more than one cavity will be opened simultaneously). There is a risk of aggravating hypothermia, and underwarmer bedding may be helpful, but the best way to mitigate for hypothermia is a warm environment (30°C). This will feel too hot for the surgeon but is better for the patient. In addition, it will serve as a constant reminder to the surgeon to abbreviate the surgery!

Equipment includes a major laparotomy set, major vascular and thoracotomy equipment. Additional equipment includes blood and blood product storage facilities, level 1 blood warmer, x-ray (fluoroscopy) equipment and occasionally a cell saver device to reuse the patient's own blood. Most important, 20 large abdominal packs must be available within the surgical field and already accounted for (nursing pre-count) and ready to use. These are placed by the scrub nurse within easy reach of the surgeon.

Patient position

The patient is placed supine on the operating table in a T-shape configuration with the arms outstretched (*crucifix position*) (**Figure 8.1**). The patient is draped from the neck to

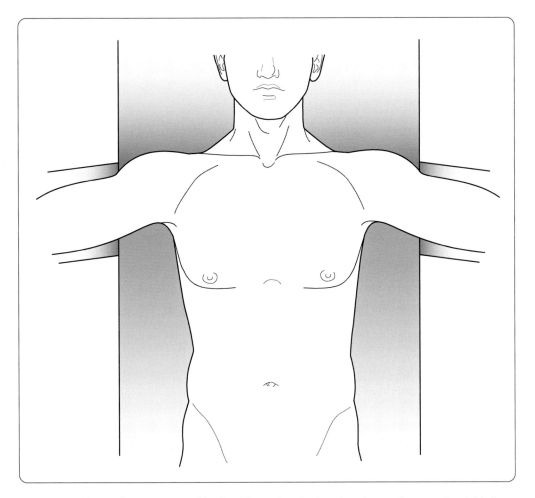

Figure 8.1 Trauma laparotomy positioning. The patient is placed supine on the operating table in a T-shape configuration with the arms outstretched.

the knees with as much lateral exposure as possible. Large bore multichannel central venous line and bladder catheters may be placed, but if *in extremis*, these may be deferred until later as long as there are at least two working wide-bore IV lines in place. The pre-operative World Health Organization (WHO) checklist must also be deferred (or abbreviated) if the patient is *in extremis*.

The technique

Remember, the clock is ticking and the surgeon must decide as he/she makes the first incision whether this is going to be an abbreviated damage control trauma laparotomy from the outset or a standard trauma laparotomy without the need for damage control manoeuvres. If DCS is indicated, a certain tempo must be maintained, remaining cognisant of rapid gross haemorrhage and contamination control followed by early termination of surgery.

The incision

Figure 8.2a follows the same procedure as any standard emergency laparotomy, but the abdominal wall is opened along its full length with the surgical knife only and in about four sweeps of the blade (and not electrocautery, which is slower). The linea alba is incised and entry into the abdomen proceeds taking care not to damage bowel which is often floating within the haemoperitoneum.

Once inside

If a massive haemoperitoneum is encountered, don't panic! The blood is already outside of the patient's intravascular space. The best first manoeuvre is to exteriorise (eviscerate) the small bowel in its entirety by sweeping it from the left side of the abdominal cavity outwards (**Figure 8.2b**). This will assist in stemming any major mesenteric bleeding (albeit temporarily) as the base of the mesentery is tamponaded against the patient's open right side abdominal wall. It also permits access for packing into the left abdominal cavity. Rolled large abdominal packs are placed sequentially, starting at the left upper quadrant (the spleen is statistically the most prevalent compelling source of bleeding in a blind trauma laparotomy), left paracolic gutter and intraperitoneal pelvic cavity (i.e. moving in a clockwise fashion) (**Figure 8.2c**). The small bowel is then re-mobilised to overhang the left side of the patient's open abdominal wall and the same packing procedure is followed in the right side of the abdominal cavity, the right side of the intraperitoneal pelvic cavity, the right paracolic gutter and the right upper quadrant (above, below and lateral to the liver) (**Figure 8.2d**). Additional packs may then be placed centrally overlying the retroperitoneum, in the superior and inferior aspects (supra- and inframesocolic spaces) and the small bowel and mesentery. The small bowel is then replaced back into the abdomen centrally. A large abdominal swab is then placed on top of the small bowel (now back *in situ*) and the surgeon places his hands on top of this and compresses gently downwards, placing moderate pressure on the abdominal contents. Then stop and wait!

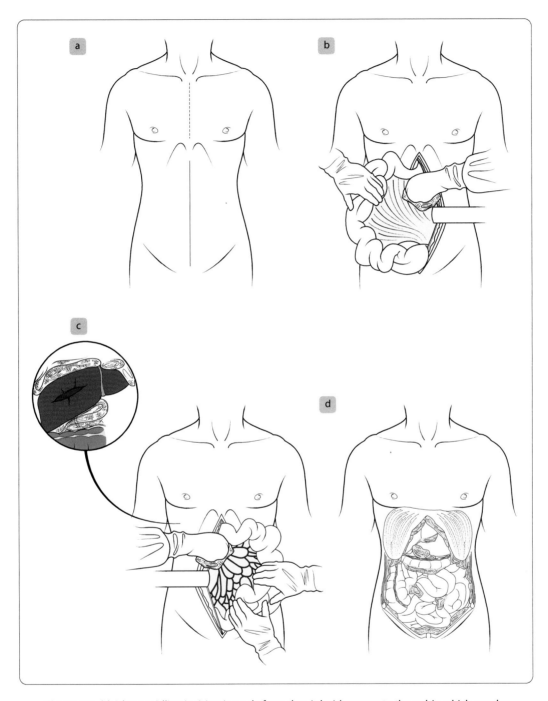

Figure 8.2 (a) A long midline incision is made from the xiphoid process to the pubis, which may be extended into the chest (and further) if necessary. (b) Exteriorise the small bowel from the duodenojejunal (DJ) flexure to the ileocolic peritoneum. Packing begins in the left upper quadrant, left paracolic gutter and intraperitoneal pelvic cavity. (c) The small bowel is mobilised to overhang over the left abdominal wall and the process is repeated in the right hand side of the abdominal cavity and up to the liver. Packs are placed in the right upper quadrant above and below the right lobe of the liver. (d) More packs are then placed in the central part of the abdomen in the superior and inferior aspect and the small bowel and mesentery returned to the abdominal cavity and pressure placed on top. Then stop and wait!

Then what?

The surgeon waits and communicates with the anaesthetic team to assess the haemodynamic response and haematological parameters. This *pause period* also allows the anaesthetic team to 'catch up' with resuscitation (now that gross haemorrhage control has been achieved) using blood and blood products (but limited crystalloid). The patient's parameters are continually reassessed by both the surgeon and the anaesthetic team. If possible, a blood gas should be sent (if not already) to assess the acid-base status and the temperature should be under continuous monitoring. The surgeon (in conjunction with the whole team) may then decide if abbreviated damage control surgery is indicated (if this was not already decided prior to 'knife-to-skin'). The surgeon and team must remain vigilant to the changing parameters and patient's dynamic condition and be prepared to change the planned surgical track in response to the changing situation.

One pitfall is that the packs are removed too early, thereby aggravating bleeding that is potentially under control. Resist this temptation! If the bleeding has been controlled and a brief but adequate period of reassessment has taken place, we advocate removal of the packs in a sequential manner beginning at the area least likely injured or bleeding. By doing this, the surgeon can declare these areas in sequence as 'injury free' thereby allowing him/her to concentrate on the more severely injured parts of the abdomen.

Total haemorrhage control

If there is continuing or uncontrolled bleeding (typically arterial) after packing (this may not be appreciated at first if the patient is very hypotensive), then a more definitive procedure may need to be performed. *Total haemorrhage control* of arterial inflow to the abdomen is typically reserved for uncontrolled or uncontrollable haemorrhage (typically seen with larger arterial injuries such as the aorta) or patients *in extremis*. This is performed by compressing the supra-coeliac aorta (typically manually at first, i.e. the aorta squeezed between the thumb and index finger) or a pressure device applied against the aorta (e.g. aortic stop device) to compress it against the thoracic vertebrae, followed by application of a supracoeliac vascular clamp (if the surgeon's skills and experience allow).

The supracoeliac aorta (i.e. the aorta above the visceral segment) is accessed by pulling the stomach downwards (caudal direction), identifying the gastrohepatic ligament (lesser omentum) and opening a window in this ligament (preferably at its medial aspect), which allows the surgeon direct access onto the aorta as it passes through the diaphragmatic aortic hiatus. This can be a challenging manoeuvre even in experienced hands and especially when time is critical. If a vascular clamp is applied, first the surgeon must sweep the intra-abdominal portion of the oesophagus away from the aorta towards the patient's left side. Failure to do this risks injuring the oesophagus (often missed!) and failure to adequately clamp the aorta. The right and left crus of the diaphragm must also be divided, as they overlay tethered to the aorta. Occasionally this may be done with manual and digital dissection, but more typically, the diaphragmatic crus must be split with scissors. Failure to split the crus and strip it from the aorta risks inadequate clamping of the aorta itself or a risk of the clamp inadvertently slipping off after application.

A preferred option for the patient *in extremis* in need of immediate and total arterial inflow control to the abdomen is to perform a left antero-lateral (or clamshell) thoracotomy, followed by immediate cross-clamping of the descending thoracic aorta as described in Chapter 4. In addition, the intra-thoracic inferior vena cava (IVC) may also be accessed and clamped from the left chest, with total loss of venous return to the heart (warn the anaesthetic team and resuscitate aggressively through IV lines above the level of the diaphragm).

Other abdominal manoeuvres

Many of these are discussed in more detail in Chapter 9 'Abdominal Trauma'. As reiterated before, this is damage control surgery and the most important goal is to stop the haemorrhage and contain the sepsis. If the packs are grossly controlling the haemorrhage, then there is no urgency to remove them. It may be best to leave *in situ* until the next phase of damage control surgery begins.

Massive bleeding typically originates from the spleen, liver, peri-pancreatic or the major vessels of the retroperitoneum (aorta, IVC and their branches). If massive bleeding is from the spleen, then a splenectomy is indicated (see Chapter 9). We *do not advocate any role for splenic preservation* in this situation. If massive bleeding is from the liver, divide the falciform ligament and re-constitute the normal anatomical shape of the liver manually by applying bimanual compression. This is followed by packing the liver firmly into its normal anatomical shape and within its normal liver bed (see Chapter 9). Other manoeuvres for managing liver bleeding, including hepatic vascular inflow control (Pringle manoeuvre), are also discussed in Chapter 9.

If an aortic injury is suspected, this will typically require aortic clamping initially either *via* the supracoeliac approach as described in the 'Total haemorrhage control' section (above) or *via* the chest (Chapter 4). Once initial massive haemorrhage is controlled, the clamp may be readjusted and repositioned as appropriate (including to the infra-renal aorta, which is preferable to restore mesenteric and renal perfusion).

Aortic injuries below the level of the mesocolon may be approached in the standard fashion for abdominal aortic aneurysm surgery (i.e. infra-mesocolic dissection and opening of the retroperitoneum below the level of the renal arteries). The ligament of Treitz is dissected and mobilised to allow the duodenum and small bowel to be swept towards the right side of the abdomen. The peritoneum is picked up and opened to allow dissection directly on to the aorta for safe clamping. Aortic injuries above the mesocolon (i.e. supramesocolic or at/above the level of the renal arteries) or where the surgeon is unsure of the position of injury require exposure *via* the *left medial visceral rotation* (Mattox manoeuvre) (Chapter 9).

Massive bleeding from an IVC injury may be initially controlled with direct pressure (low-pressure, high-flow vessel), but is best exposed *via* the *right medial visceral rotation* (Cattell–Braasch manoeuvre), which is further discussed in Chapter 9.

The retroperitoneum

The retroperitoneum (RP) is carefully inspected for haematoma. A zone 1 (midzone) RP haematoma must be explored, including if seen on CT scan, regardless of whether the mechanism was blunt or penetrating. A zone 2 RP haematoma (i.e. lateral around the kidneys) should be explored if it is expanding or pulsatile intra-operatively, as this indicates an arterial bleed (most venous bleeds will tamponade spontaneously surrounded by

Gerota's fascia). Remember, an arterial extravasation 'blush' seen on computed tomography is a radiological equivalent of an arterial bleed or expanding haematoma and mandates exploration. In addition, maintain a low threshold for exploring a zone 2 RP haematoma after all penetrating injuries to this zone (even if the haematoma is non-pulsatile and non-expanding), as there is a higher likelihood of an injury requiring surgery (e.g. renal calyx), including a subtle injury to the posterior wall of the ascending/descending colon respectively. Finally, a zone 3 RP (i.e. the pelvis below the peritoneal reflection) injury should only be entered if it is expanding or pulsatile, but also maintain a low threshold for surgical exploration after a penetrating injury due to the high likelihood of injury to one of the pelvic organs.

Hollow viscus injury

Small holes in the small bowel may be closed primarily in a transverse or circular fashion to prevent stenosis. Severely damaged small bowel should be rapidly oversewn or resected to manage contamination and the ends stapled closed (or tied with a heavy suture/tape). The bowel may be left in discontinuity for a number of days, as typically there will be an ileus anyway. In addition, any attempt to anastomose in the face of profound shock and damage control is likely to lead to dehiscence and further sepsis (second-hit phenomenon).

Other important injuries not to miss

All other injuries require a full exploratory laparotomy if physiology allows. The most likely locations of missed injuries (which must be inspected and ruled out directly and specifically) are

- Gastro-oesophageal junction
- Anterior and posterior wall of the stomach
- Pancreas and duodenum (anterior and posterior aspects)
- Transverse colon
- Ascending and descending colon
- Root of the mesentery
- Rectum

At the end of damage control surgery stage I

The abdomen is typically left open with the packs *in situ*, but if the patient is *in extremis*, use a running suture to close the skin only (leave the fascial domain untouched for definitive repair later) to enhance the abdominal tamponade and gross haemorrhage control. This is superior to other temporary closure methods (e.g. Bogota bag sutured to the aponeurosis) so as to preserve the oedematous aponeurosis, in addition to being a time-consuming procedure. If relatively stable at this point, or if the skin cannot be approximated, we advise fashioning a laparostomy with vacuum dressing, which may be either improvised using Ioban™ and surgical swabs or if available, using a commercially available device (e.g. Abthera™).

The patient is then returned to the ICU for aggressive management of the metabolic derangements and reversal of the coagulopathy, hypothermia and acidosis, reversal of haemodynamic disruption, adequate intravascular filling (blood and blood products and limited crystalloid) and further management and diagnosis of any potentially missed injury (especially TBI and spine). The aim of DCS stage II is to prepare the patient for a return to the operating suite for the relook procedure and perhaps definitive management of injuries, assessment of potentially missed injuries and definitive closure of the abdomen (if appropriate). The patient must have enough restored physiological and metabolic reserve for this next stage in their journey and to withstand further surgical insult.

We would advocate aiming for DCS stage III as soon as possible, but typically this will take place at about 24–48 hours after the index operation. Occasionally the take back may be after 72 hours, but it is not ideal to leave the packs *in situ* longer than this as they begin to become infected and septic with the risk of a further inflammatory insult (i.e. second-hit phenomenon) which the patient may not recover from. Ensure all packs are accounted for on removal, then toilet the abdominal cavity with copious amounts of warm saline and drain the abdomen widely. The abdomen may then be closed definitively (although some advocate leaving the skin open for an additional 48 hours to avoid a superficial wound infection). If the abdominal domain cannot be closed tension free, then a staged procedure is indicated (beyond the scope of this chapter). Continue to monitor these patients for the development of abdominal compartment syndrome after successful closure.

Additional reading

Bowley DM, Barker P, Boffard KD. Damage control surgery – Concepts and practice. *J R Army Med Corps* 2000;146(3):176–182.

Brasel KJ, Weigelt JA. Damage control in trauma surgery. *Curr Opin Crit Care* 2000;6(4):276–280.

Cirocchi R, Abraha I, Montedori A et al. Damage control surgery for abdominal trauma. *Cochrane Database Syst Rev* 2010(1):CD007438.

Diaz JJ Jr., Cullinane DC, Dutton WD et al. The management of the open abdomen in trauma and emergency general surgery: Part 1 – Damage control. *J Trauma* 2010;68(6):1425–1438.

Duchesne JC, Kimonis K, Marr AB et al. Damage control resuscitation in combination with damage control laparotomy: A survival advantage. *J Trauma* 2010;69(1):46–52.

Eiseman B, Moore EE, Meldrum DR, Raeburn C. Feasibility of damage control surgery in the management of military combat casualties. *Arch Surg* 2000;135(11):1323–1327.

Goldberg SR, Henning J, Wolfe LG, Duane TM. Practice patterns for the use of antibiotic agents in damage control laparotomy and its impact on outcomes. *Surg Infect (Larchmt)* 2017;18(3):282–286.

Hirshberg A, Walden R. Damage control for abdominal trauma. *Surg Clin North Am* 1997;77(4):813–820.

Hommes M, Chowdhury S, Visconti D et al. Contemporary damage control surgery outcomes: 80 patients with severe abdominal injuries in the right upper quadrant analyzed. *Eur J Trauma Emerg Surg* 2018;44(1):79–85.

Karamarkovic AR, Popovic NM, Blagojevic ZB et al. Damage control surgery in abdominal trauma. *Acta Chir Iugosl* 2010;57(1):15–24.

Kirkpatrick AW, McKee JL, Tien H et al. Damage control surgery in weightlessness: A comparative study of simulated torso hemorrhage control comparing terrestrial and weightless conditions. *J Trauma Acute Care Surg* 2017;82(2):392–399.

Moore EE, Burch JM, Franciose RJ, Offner PJ, Biffl WL. Staged physiologic restoration and damage control surgery. *World J Surg* 1998;22(12):1184–1190; discussion 1190–1191.

Morgan K, Mansker D, Adams DB. Not just for trauma patients: Damage control laparotomy in pancreatic surgery. *J Gastrointest Surg* 2010;14(5):768–772.

Myrhoj T, Moller P. Liver packing and planned reoperation in the management of severe hepatic trauma. *Annales Chirurgiae et Gynaecologiae* 1987;76(4):215–217.

Parajuli P, Kumar S, Gupta A et al. Role of laparoscopy in patients with abdominal trauma at level-I trauma center. *Surg Laparosc Endosc Percutan Tech* 2018;28(1):20–25.

Poortman P, Meeuwis JD, Leenen LP. [Multitrauma patients: Principles of 'damage control surgery']. *Ned Tijdschr Geneeskd* 2000;144(28):1337–1341.

Rignault DP. Abdominal trauma in war. *World J Surg* 1992;16(5):940–946.

Rotondo MF, Schwab CW, McGonigal MD et al. 'Damage control': An approach for improved survival in exsanguinating penetrating abdominal injury. *J Trauma* 1993;35(3):375–382; discussion 382–383.

Scalea TM, Phillips TF, Goldstein AS et al. Injuries missed at operation: Nemesis of the trauma surgeon. *J Trauma* 1988;28(7):962–967.

Schellenberg M, Inaba K, Bardes JM et al. Defining the GE junction in trauma: Epidemiology and management of a challenging injury. *J Trauma Acute Care Surg* 2017;83(5):798–802.

Smith JE, Midwinter M, Lambert AW. Avoiding cavity surgery in penetrating torso trauma: The role of the computed tomography scan. *Ann R Coll Surg Engl* 2010;92(6):486–488.

Sharrock AE, Barker T, Yuen HM, Rickard R, Tai N. Management and closure of the open abdomen after damage control laparotomy for trauma. A systematic review and meta-analysis. *Injury* 2016;47(2):296–306.

Timmermans J, Nicol A, Kairinos N, Teijink J, Prins M, Navsaria P. Predicting mortality in damage control surgery for major abdominal trauma. *S Afr J Surg* 2010;48(1):6–9.

Zacharias SR, Offner P, Moore EE, Burch J. Damage control surgery. *AACN Clin Issues* 1999;10(1):95–103; quiz 141–142.

9 Abdominal Trauma

Mansoor Khan

Introduction

Statistically, abdominal trauma is the most prevalent compelling source of bleeding in the haemodynamically unstable, severely injured patient and management often includes performing a 'blind' (in the absence of advanced diagnostic studies) trauma laparotomy, for both diagnosis and/or treatment. Even patients who present relatively well after trauma, the abdomen can still provide unique diagnostic challenges including 'missed injuries' and/or delayed interventions for subtle intra-abdominal trauma, which are associated with a higher morbidity and mortality, from a combination of blood loss and GI spillage. Mechanism of abdominal injury includes blunt and penetrating, which follow the same initial assessment and management as other injuries, excepting immediate transfer to theatre for emergency laparotomy in the exsanguinating patient.

Vehicular crashes are a common cause of blunt abdominal injury (spleen, liver and small bowel in descending order). Although the associated incidence of traumatic brain injury (TBI) and significant thoracic trauma have decreased over time with seat belt usage and enhancements in vehicular safety, there has been a comparative rise in the prevalence of isolated seat belt–induced abdominal trauma. Many of these patients (who historically would have died prehospital) are now more likely to arrive in hospital alive, but with an intra-abdominal (perhaps initially subtle) injury requiring intervention.

Penetrating abdominal trauma (stabbings, GSW, etc) often presents with a visually 'minor' external wound, creating a diagnostic challenge in the haemodynamically well patient with regards to peritoneal cavity breach (higher incidence of significant intra-abdominal organ injury with peritoneal breach).

The biggest challenge managing complex polytrauma is deciding the order of cavity (chest, abdomen or pelvis) exploration, or if at all (i.e. where is the most compelling source of haemorrhage?). It is wholly acceptable to blindly explore the abdomen if there is *any* suspicion of significant injury. Statistically, significant bleeding is most prevalent in the abdomen and a 'blind laparotomy' is also a diagnostic manoeuvre as well as being potentially therapeutic. Therefore, we do not use the term 'negative laparotomy,' preferring to advocate for a *non-therapeutic diagnostic laparotomy* for those patients who undergo surgery and in whom no significant injury is found. Such an approach has not been shown to increase mortality in the polytrauma patient and although there may be an associated morbidity with any laparotomy, these complications are insignificant compared with a missed injury which can be devastating. In addition, a low 'missed injury rate' is an independent metric in a mature, well-functioning trauma system.

Always assume the patient is sick, until they prove to you that they are well

Professor Thomas Scalea
Physician-in-chief
R Adams Cowley Shock Trauma Center
Baltimore, Maryland, USA

Working anatomy for trauma

The abdominal cavity is a *non-compressible cavity*, surrounded by the anterior and posterior walls (joined at the flanks), and superiorly by the diaphragm (junctional zone with the thorax) and inferiorly by the pelvis (junctional zone) which will also accommodate significant haemorrhage (**Figure 9.1**).

For the purposes of identifying the source of abdominal bleeding, subdivide the cavities into the following compartments for exploration:

1. *Intraperitoneal compartment* – This is the true peritoneal cavity bounded superiorly by the diaphragm and lower rib cage (some protection from trauma here). This *thoraco-abdominal region* (junctional zone) contains the liver, spleen, stomach and transverse colon. The section above the transverse colon is the *supracolic compartment* containing a dense population of abdominal organs and network of vessels. Haemorrhage here

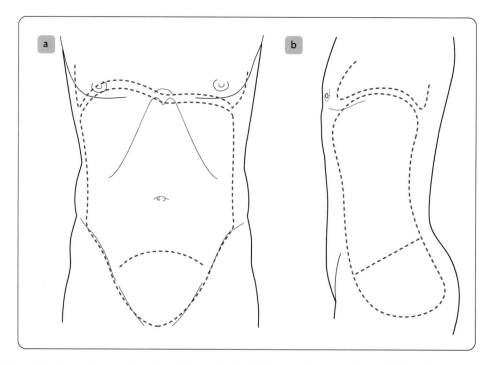

Figure 9.1 (a) The true peritoneal cavity from the front. It is a sizable cavity into which bleeding can occur with little natural tamponade. (b) Peritoneal cavity and the potential space for bleeding as seen from the side.

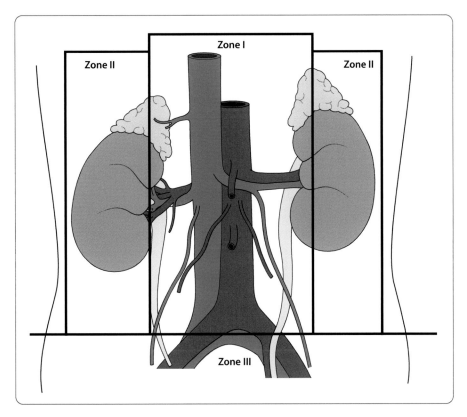

Figure 9.2 The three zones of the retroperitoneum. Zone I is the central area at the back of the abdomen, behind the parietal peritoneum and contains the major vessels including the aorta, IVC and their branches. Zone II is the lateral RP, consisting of the kidneys and ureters. Zone III is the extraperitoneal pelvic cavity (below the iliac crests).

is challenging to expose. Below the transverse colon is the *infracolic compartment* (mostly bowel).

2. *Retroperitoneal compartment* (**Figure 9.2**) – This is a potential cavity (which may be greatly enlarged with significant bleeding) at the back of the abdomen encompassing the entire posterior portion of the abdominal cavity. It is covered with a dense layer of parietal peritoneum and contains a dense vascular and fibre network of nervous plexus and connective tissue. The retroperitoneum (RP) is further divided into three broad zones, each with unique challenges.
   - **Zone I**: Central RP containing the major vascular structures and their branches including: aorta and inferior vena cava (IVC) and the pancreas in the upper segment (overlying the visceral portion of the aorta).
   - **Zone II**: This is the lateral RP out to the flanks and contains the kidneys, ureters and muscle of the posterior abdominal wall, in addition to the ascending and descending colon (both retroperitoneal).
   - **Zone III**: This is the true pelvic compartment. It is surrounded by the pelvic bones and contains a multitude of vascular structures, associated with major haemorrhage when torn (iliac arteries and accompanying veins) in addition to the pelvic organs (rectum, urinary bladder, reproductive organs).

Regions prone to devascularisation and missed injuries

There are a variety of locations within the abdomen, prone to devascularisation, especially with a deceleration-type injury. This occurs at junctions where there is an immobile–mobile interface of viscera (**Figure 9.3**). Also, there are five regions that readily house missed injuries and must be inspected individually:

- Gastro-oesophageal junction
- Anterior and posterior wall of the stomach
- Pancreas and duodenum (anterior and posterior aspects)
- Transverse colon
- Ascending and descending colon
- Root of the mesentery
- Rectum

Managing intra-abdominal injuries

This section discusses the management of individual abdominal organ injury during trauma laparotomy (Chapter 8), including supracoeliac control of the aorta.

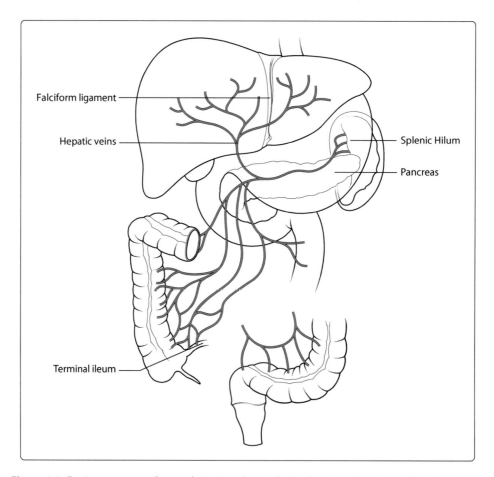

Figure 9.3 Regions prone to devascularisation due to their relative 'tethering' to other structures.

Supracoeliac control

> Your hand is an excellent haemostatic device
>
> Avoid clamping blindly

The initial approach is *as per* the description for the trauma laparotomy (Chapter 8). A long midline incision is performed with a few sweeps of the surgical knife and, once the peritoneum is open, fully eviscerate the small bowel to the patient's right hand side, packing the cavity as previously described. If correctly-performed but still does not achieve temporary haemostasis, then consider the possibility of an abdominal arterial injury. The best initial compression technique is manual compression. Open a generous window in the lesser omentum (gastro-hepatic ligament), taking care not to disrupt a potential aberrant left hepatic artery (5%–10% of the population) which arises directly from the coeliac trunk and travels transverse through the lesser omentum.

The supracoeliac aorta is palpated posteriorly in the midline against the bony spine and the intra-abdominal segment of the oesophagus at its left side. It should have a pulse present, but in the extremely shocked patient, this may not be immediately appreciated. It is also surrounded by and encased with the right and left diaphragmatic crus as it passes from the thorax into the abdomen. These are musculo-tendinous portions of the diaphragm and are tough to dissect. (**Figure 9.4**). Initially, the aorta may be pinched (between thumb and forefinger) or compressed against the bony spine with the fist. It is difficult to get complete occlusion of the aorta and the hand can become fatigued very quickly. A vascular clamp cannot be safely applied until the connective tissue and both diaphragmatic crus' have been dissected free.

For patients *in extremis* from haemorrhage with a suspected intra-abdominal source, or potential for problematic intra-abdominal control (e.g. hostile abdomen), then a *left antero-lateral thoracotomy* with cross-clamping of the descending thoracic aorta is the most rapid and effective way to gain immediate abdominal in-flow control.

Solid organ injuries

Splenic injury

Splenic trauma has gone through several accepted standards of care over the past three decades. Historically, all injured spleens were removed which was deemed the safest option due to a combination of a lack of availability of CT scanning (and thus were often discovered during laparotomy prompting removal), the risk of delayed bleeding, a poor understanding of the natural history of non-operative management (NOM) and under-developed critical care facilities. There is now good clinical evidence to support splenic preservation with NOM, sometimes misleadingly referred to as 'conservative management'. However, in order to ensure a patient is both suitable and safe for NOM of splenic trauma, certain criteria must be met: The patient must be haemodynamically normal with no peritonitis or any other indication for laparotomy. The success rate for NOM in a haemodynamically normal (most important) patient with a splenic injury is in the region of about 70% overall, with higher failure rates associated with higher grades of injury. Many experts do not

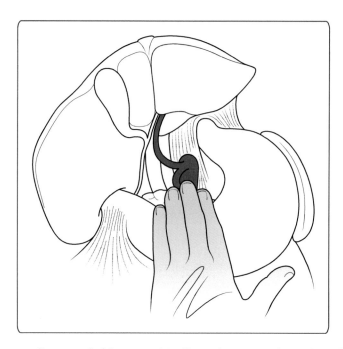

Figure 9.4 Supracoeliac control of the aorta: this effectively gives total vascular in-flow control to the abdomen. The supracoeliac aorta is palpated by dissecting through the lesser omentum (gastro-hepatic ligament) and palpating it against the midline vertebrae. Initially, manual compression may be used, but for effective and safe cross-clamping, the intra-abdominal portion of the oesophagus will need to be swept away from the aorta (towards the patient's left hand side) and the right and left diaphragmatic crus (and other connective tissue) separated from the aorta itself, with a combination of sharp and blunt dissection.

permit NOM for a grade V splenic injury regardless of the haemodynamics. In addition, some advocate empirical splenectomy for grades III – V in those patients who will poorly tolerate any complication arising during NOM (e.g. delayed rupture, abscess formation, pain and poor respiratory effort). This group also includes those with severe concurrent traumatic brain injury (TBI).

The major indications for trauma splenectomy are:

- Major haemorrhage from an injured spleen with haemodynamic compromise
- Failure of NOM for splenic injury
- Concurrent TBI (controversial)

Although operative splenic conservation (e.g. suture repair, mesh repair, etc) is well-described and advocated for, it absolutely should not be attempted in the haemodynamically compromised patient. Potential complications arising from operative splenic preservation include: re-bleeding and shock and infection/abscess formation. We do not practice or advocate operative splenic conservation for this group of patients or indeed if they have failed a trial of NOM, as a failure of NOM is an absolute indication itself to remove the spleen.

A failure of NOM includes any haemodynamic instability that occurs during a trial of NOM, as it indicates the higher likelihood that the spleen is continuing to bleed and self-tamponade has not occurred effectively. A fall in haemoglobin and/or repeated blood transfusion (even in the haemodynamically well patient) is also another indication, as it indicates continuous bleeding from the spleen and a higher likelihood of delayed rupture. Either way, if the patient fails NOM, a splenectomy (and not splenic preservation) is indicated. A concurrent TBI is a controversial indication, but many experts feel that a sudden splenic rupture with hypotension in an unacceptable risk in this patient group.

> There is no role for operative splenic preservation for the injured spleen

> A failure of non-operative management of a splenic injury is an absolute indication for splenectomy

> There is no role for splenic conservation in the physiologically or haemodynamically compromised patient

> Splenectomy is the damage control option for splenic injury

The role of interventional radiology (IR)

Interventional radiology (IR) is quickly becoming an accepted standard of care as part of the management of splenic trauma, but only in the physiologically non-compromised patient. However, this is most suitable for those patients displaying a definite contrast extravasation 'blush' on computer tomography angiography (CTA), which indicates an arterial bleed, which may then be embolised. The popularity of IR in splenic injury is that it improves the success rate for NOM when a 'blush' is present. However, most splenic bleeding is parenchymal/capillary (i.e. not arterial) and IR offers little benefit in this group over NOM alone. However, there is a growing body of evidence highlighting the complications of IR for splenic injury including splenic infarction, infection, abscess formation, sepsis and gastric infarction. Ensure these groups are selected appropriately.

Performing a splenectomy

This follows on from Chapter 8. Once packed and gross bleeding control is obtained, the packs are carefully removed to identify sources of bleeding. Start by removing packs from the areas least likely injured. Once the packs are removed from the left upper quadrant (LUQ), there will be haemorrhage and clot (the haemorrhage may be temporised due to hypotension). Often an injured spleen is manually palpated rather than seen due to its posterior position in the LUQ (**Figure 9.5**).

For best exposure, stand on the patient's right and have an assistant elevate the left lower rib cage upwards using an abdominal wall retractor (e.g. Morris retractor). Place your right hand over the spleen and deep into the LUQ along the plane between the spleen and

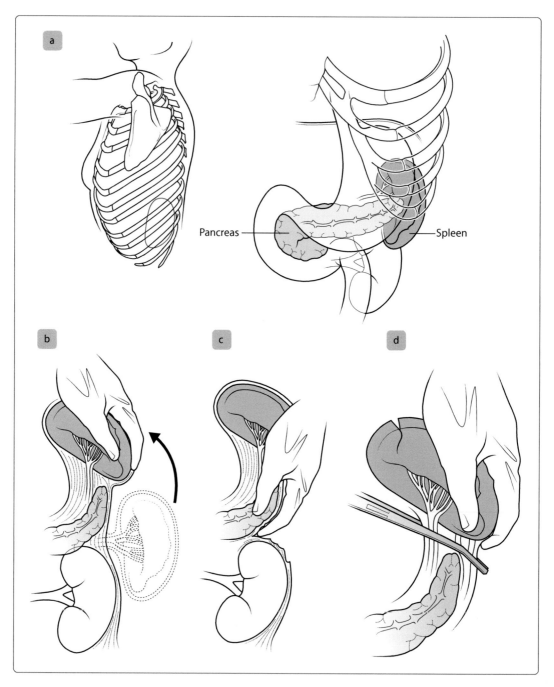

Figure 9.5 (a) Location of the spleen deep and posterior in the LUQ. (b) Mobilisation of the spleen: divide the splenophrenic and splenorenal ligaments so that the spleen may be elevated out of its natural bed and into the abdominal midline. (c) Additional manual dissection may be necessary to separate the spleen from surrounding tissue for effective elevation. Take care not to injure the tail of pancreas or the short gastric vessels. (d) Splenic hilar control. Once elevated, a vascular clamp may be safely placed across the splenic hilum for vascular control. *(Continued)*

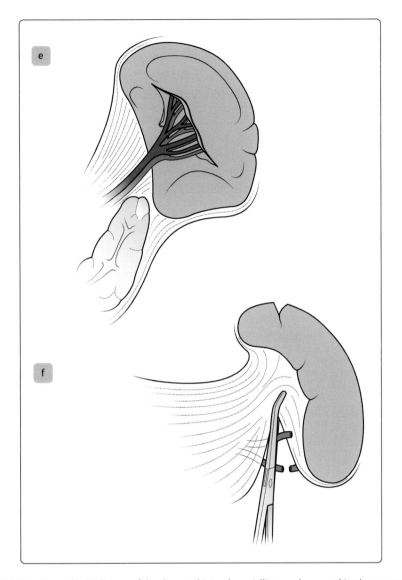

Figure 9.5 (Continued) (e) Once safely elevated into the midline and cupped in the surgeons left hand, the splenic hilum may be inspected (not always this long). (f) The short gastric vessels are divided separately (if necessary) and the tail of pancreas inspected. Ideally, ligate and divide the splenic vessels individually, but more typically the splenic hilum is clamped, the spleen removed and the hilum transfixed *en masse*.

the abdominal wall, in an attempt to separate the organ from its bed. Elevate it into the midline of the open abdomen (i.e. mobilise it from its lateral plane of dissection). *Make the spleen a midline organ.* The various peritoneal attachments (e.g. lienophrenic, splenorenal, lienocolic, splenophrenic ligaments) are typically already shattered and torn, and most of the dissection has already been done by the haematoma. In this case, attempt to elevate the shattered spleen as a whole into the midline. If the peritoneal attachments are still partially intact, then they may be separated manually with blunt dissection, but occasionally sharp dissection and division is necessary.

As the right hand elevates the injured spleen into the midline (more difficult if splenomegaly is present), then place it into your left hand (i.e. cup it in the left hand with the splenic hilum structures placed between the left index and middle fingers and compress the vessels between the digits to control bleeding). The tail of the pancreas is often also elevated with the spleen and care must be taken not to injure it in addition (**Figure 9.5a–f**).

Note: Back-bleeding may continue from the short gastric vessels. Once elevated, place large abdominal packs into the splenic bed behind within the LUQ to prevent the spleen falling back, in addition to tamponading any haemorrhage within the LUQ from the dissection. A vascular clamp may then be applied to the splenic hilum, taking care to avoid the short gastric vessels (unless these too are also bleeding) and avoid injuring the distal pancreatic tail.

Once the hilum is controlled, ideally each major splenic vessel should be individually identified and ligated separately. However, this isn't typically possible with complete shatter of the hilum or in the haemodynamically compromised patient, in which case the entire splenic hilum may be suture-ligated *en masse*, followed by division of the hilum and removal of the spleen. An additional running suture may be necessary if there is continued bleeding from the remaining ligated hilar tissue. The short gastric vessels (variable position) may require separate and individual ligation, taking care not to damage the greater curvature of the stomach (or identify and repair it if injury has occurred).

For the patient is *in extremis*, place an aortic clamp across the hilum and remove the spleen by dividing the hilum distal to the clamp.

Occasionally a very enlarged spleen is proving too difficult to safely mobilise to the midline to gain hilar control. In this circumstance, it may be preferable to ligate the splenic artery at the coeliac plexus. This will cause the spleen to shrink and allow easier dissection and delivery.

Hepatic injury

The liver is the second most commonly injured intra-abdominal organ in blunt trauma. Compared with splenic injury however, the success rate for hepatic injury NOM in appropriately selected cases is much higher (>85%). However, if surgery is required, liver injuries can be much more complex to manage (obviously it cannot be simply removed!). Thankfully, the majority of liver injuries encountered during trauma laparotomy require minimal intervention with excellent outcomes.

When operative management is required, it is typically for higher-grade injuries, although lower-grade injuries can bleed extensively on occasion and management is almost always damage control. However, for high-grade liver injuries we advise a *'less is more'* approach in damage control, as any attempts at heroic manoeuvres will almost always end with the demise of the severely injured patient.

Hepatic mobilisation and dissection should be kept to a minimum if circumstances allow

Operative management

This follows on from Chapter 8, where a trauma laparotomy and damage control abdominal packing has already taken place for gross haemorrhage control.

Initial operative management

The injured liver must be packed in to its normal anatomical shape where possible and into its normal liver bed. To achieve this, the falciform ligament must be taken down (i.e. clamped, divided and ligated), which is already part of the normal trauma laparotomy. This allows access to the liver and reduces the risk of iatrogenic injury (relatively fixed point on the liver). Your hands are probably the best initial tool to manually compress the fractured liver back together by attempting to approximate its torn edges into the normal (i.e. pre-injury) anatomical shape (i.e. restore normal hepatic anatomy with bimanual compression). As the majority of liver bleeding is venous-pressure only (hepatic and portal veins), this will temporise most haemorrhage. It is important to remember that while doing this, do not be tempted to pack inside a liver laceration, no matter how large. This will only force the liver parenchyma further apart with more tearing and bleeding, and will fail to create the required tamponade.

At the same time, manually compress the liver backwards into the liver bed in the right upper quadrant (RUQ). In order to maintain this temporised bleeding control, use rolled up large abdominal packs to 'pack' the liver to maintain the reconstituted shape and pressure. Pack above (between liver and diaphragm), below, laterally and medially (**Figure 9.6**). Do not pack behind the liver, as this requires mobilising the liver forwards (which takes time and has a higher complication rate), which may disrupt a contained retro-hepatic haematoma

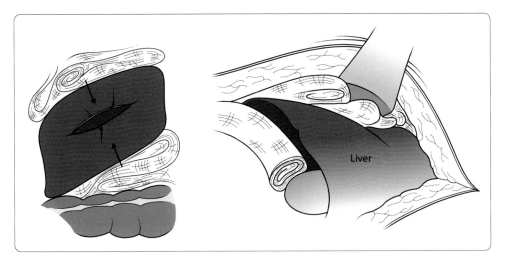

Figure 9.6 Hepatic packing. As the majority of hepatic bleeds are low pressure / capillary bleeding, most are manageable with external compression in the form of hepatic packing. Ensure the liver is compressed into its normal anatomical shape (and within its normal liver bed in the RUQ). Place rolled up large surgical swabs above, below and anterior to the liver to maintain this shape and external compression (arrows). The right triangular ligament may have to be dissected free to ensure effective lateral packing. Do not pack behind the liver as this may de-roof a stable retrohepatic haematoma.

(and possibly a retro-hepatic IVC injury). Instead, manually push the liver backwards into its bed and pack in front to effect posterior compression. Be careful not to overpack or overcompress the liver (especially the IVC), which will decrease venous return to the heart and further compromise the already shocked patient. The majority of liver bleeding will stop with these techniques, and assuming no other injuries are in need of attention, the surgeon may complete the damage control laparotomy and progress to DCS stage II.

> Aim to pack the injured liver into its normal anatomical shape and into its normal anatomical bed

> Do not pack inside hepatic lacerations

If necessary, the **Pringle manoeuvre** is necessary to gain additional hepatic inflow control (see next section).

Specific liver techniques and manoeuvres

The Pringle manoeuvre

The *Pringle manoeuvre* controls the hepatic vascular inflow. The portal vein supplies about 75% of hepatic perfusion and the hepatic artery the remaining 25% (but with equal amounts of hepatic O_2). Both of these vessels are found within the free edge of the lesser omentum (the gastro-hepatic ligament) in addition to the common bile duct (CBD): portal vein posterior and CBD and hepatic artery in front. This is manually palpated by sliding the left index finger into the *foramen of Winslow* (just below the liver) which is the natural anatomic opening to the lesser sac.

The free edge is initially pinched between the left index finger and thumb or a small window may be opened in the lesser omentum (medial to the structures to avoid damaging them) and a sling looped around them for control (**Figure 9.7**). A vascular clamp (or Rummel tourniquet) may be used to control the hepatic blood supply at this level. In elective surgery, the Pringle manoeuvre may be kept *in situ* for about 50 minutes (assuming normal liver function) before irreversible hepatic ischaemia occurs. It is not clear how long it may be kept *in situ* in the shocked polytrauma patient, but assume it is a lot shorter than 50 minutes.

Hepatic finger fracture

The hepatic finger fracture is the technique of bluntly dissecting into an actively bleeding deep liver laceration to directly visualise and ligate small bleeding vessels (especially arterial) (**Figure 9.8a**). The torn vessels are identified as small bleeding points that may be picked up with a surgical clip and ligated. The index finger of the right hand gently, but firmly 'scratches' into the laceration to separate the liver parenchyma until the spurting artery is identified and subsequently ligated. The tissues are friable and easily separated digitally to allow identification of the vessels and bile ducts. It is typically not necessary for a venous bleed, as compression alone will likely temporise this due to the lower pressure.

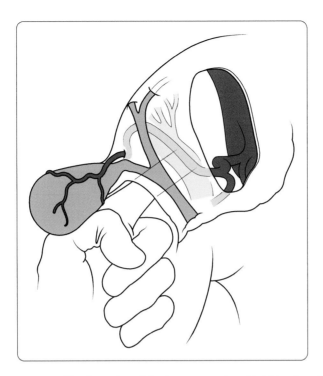

Figure 9.7 Pringle manoeuvre. The free edge of the lesser omentum (right border of the gastro-hepatic ligament) carries the three principal structures leading to the liver porta hepatis: the portal vein (behind), the common bile duct (and common hepatic duct) and the hepatic artery. Thus the entire hepatic perfusion inflow may be controlled here, by passing a finger behind this free edge of lesser omentum (i.e. through the foramen of Winslow into the lesser sac) and pinching the structures in the free edge. Make a small window in the lesser omentum, taking care not to injure these structure and pass a Rummel tourniquet around them, or use a soft bowel or vascular clamp to occlude.

Hepatic tractotomy

Hepatic tractotomy (**Figure 9.8b**) has been described for penetrating through-and-through liver injuries that create a tubular defect that is actively bleeding. If not too deep within the liver tissue (but too deep for finger fracture), a tractotomy may be performed using a linear stapler inserted into the tract and 'fired', thereby 'opening-up' the tract and exposing the bleeding vessels within. These bleeding small vessels may then be ligated or oversewn and/or an omental pedicle plug inserted into the raw surface of the tract and approximated using deep liver suturing as described below.

Deep liver (pledgeted) suture repair

Large, visibly bleeding lacerations on the liver surface may be managed with deep suturing (i.e. liver suturing). Use a brained absorbable suture (less likely to 'cheese wire' through the liver (Glisson's) capsule compared with a non-braided suture) on a large curved needle (**Figure 9.9**).

Begin the insertion point of the needle at 90° to the liver and 1–2 cm back from the laceration edge. Follow the natural curve of the needle deep through the liver parenchyma and exit on the opposite side, again about 1–2 cm from the laceration edge. Gently approximate the opposing edges of the laceration together, taking care to prevent cheese wiring of the suture through Glisson's capsule. Pledgets may also be used with the suture to prevent this

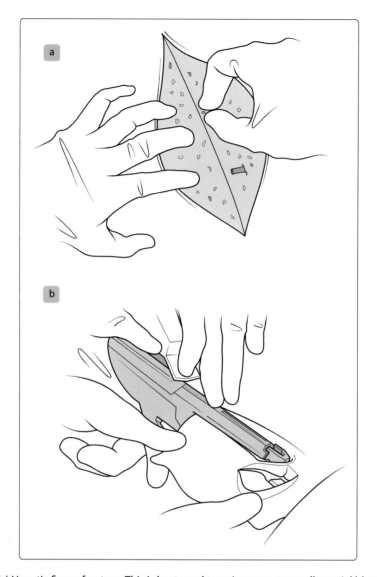

Figure 9.8 (a) Hepatic finger fracture. This is best used to gain access to small arterial bleeders deeper (but not too deep) inside a liver laceration. The index finger 'scratches' at the liver parenchyma within the liver laceration, bluntly dissecting through the tissue until the small arterial bleeders are seen, picked up and ligated. (b) Hepatic tractotomy. For relatively superficial through-and-through liver injuries, a GIA stapling device may be inserted through the tract, closed and 'fired', thereby resecting the injured segment whilst also being haemostatic. Any on-going ooze may be reinforced and oversewn after resection.

by offering additional resistance during approximation and spreading the pressure more evenly along the edge of the liver laceration. Ensure good tissue bites are taken to effect apposition of the tissue edges and therefore good haemostasis (**Figure 9.9**).

Hepatic omental plugging

This is used in conjunction with deep liver suturing (described above), typically for even deeper lacerations or where the lacerated liver edges cannot be opposed safely without

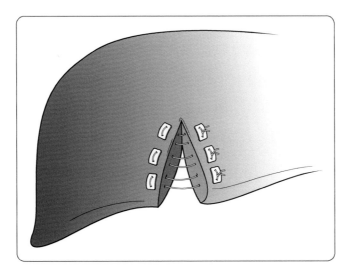

Figure 9.9 Apposition repair of liver lacerations. A braided (e.g. vicryl) suture on a large curved blunt needle is used to deeply traverse the liver parenchyma on either side of a laceration, afterwhich the edges are gently apposed and ligated to effect haemostasis within the tract of the injury. Using pledgets in addition will further reduce the risk of tissue shearing.

tearing. A free-tongue or pedicle of viable omentum is mobilised (preserving its blood supply), and 'packed' deep into the recess of the liver laceration as a 'plug' for haemostasis, which in turn fills the liver defect (**Figure 9.10**). Deep liver suturing is then utilised to gain further compression of the laceration edges against the omental plug and to hold the omental plug *in situ*. This is an excellent haemostatic adjunct which prevents dead space formation (and subsequent infection) and reduces the risk of bile leak. In circumstances where the omentum is not substantial enough for a plug, the falciform ligament may be mobilised and used for the same purpose.

Hepatic balloon tamponade

Hepatic balloon tamponade has been described for deeper through-and-through penetrating injuries (e.g. gunshot wound) that are too deep to reach with either the finger fracture technique or hepatic tractotomy. Insert a Foley catheter into a finger segment of a sterile glove and tie the proximal end closed to prevent leakage. Gently insert the gloved tip of the catheter into the traumatic liver track as far as it will comfortably go. Once inside, infuse sterile saline directly into the outer opening of the Foley catheter (not its balloon) to inflate the rubber of the glove like a balloon. This will tamponade bleeding within the trajectory tract, without having to open it up (potentially destabilising it).

Resectional debridement

Resectional debridement is generally not recommended at the index operation, as it is an added surgical burden on the already-compromised patient. It is very unusual (and unnecessary) to have to perform a formal (anatomical) lobar resection. Non-anatomical resections are more likely (if required at all), typically as a combination of finger fracture, diathermy and linear staplers, with debridement back to viable tissue. If required, it is better to perform during stage III.

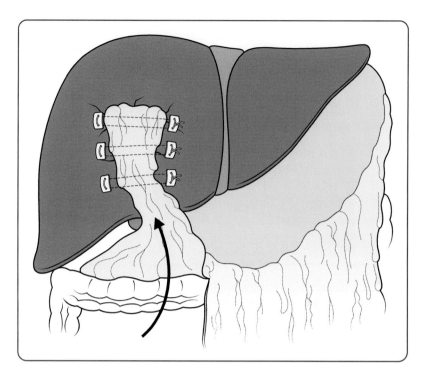

Figure 9.10 Omental hepatic pack. This is best used in a large hepatic laceration, where the edges cannot be approximated and externally compressed effectively. It is often used after the hepatic finger fracture technique and ligation of small arterial bleeding vessels, where a larger liver rent has been created. Dissect and elevate a segment of viable omentum, but leaving its blood supply intact. Place the omental pedicle into the liver laceration to fill the space. Then use deep liver sutures to gently approximate the edges or to maintain the omental pediclae in place. Pledgets may also be used with the liver sutures to prevent 'cheese wiring' through the liver capsule. The addition of the omental plug will aid in reducing a bile leak in addition to being a haemostatic manoeuvre.

Angiographic intervention

High-grade liver injuries that require damage control surgery or injuries deep inside the liver parenchyma, not safely accessible with open surgery, should undergo immediate post-operative IR (CTA first if physiology allows). A hybrid suite is the ideal location for these patients, so that transportation may be minimised. Any deep liver arterial contrast extravasation 'blush' seen, may be embolised for further haemorrhage control. There is also a high prevalence of arteriovenous (AV) fistula and pseudoaneurysm formation when a contrast 'blush' is present after trauma as well as the risk of serious iatrogenic injury if managed with open surgery.

Advanced liver techniques

Liver mobilisation

Occasionally the liver must be further mobilised to manage an injury at a difficult-to-reach position (e.g. lateral liver edge or posterior). Caution is advised if a retro-hepatic IVC injury is suspected, as mobilisation can quickly lead to loss of tamponade and rapid exsanguination.

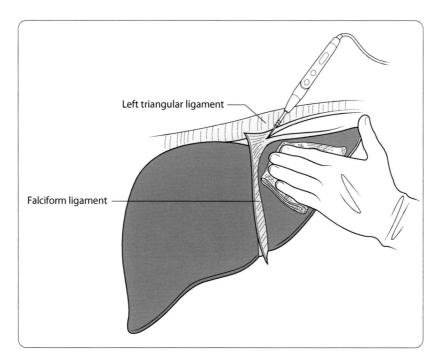

Figure 9.11 Mobilising the left lobe of liver. After ligation and division of the falciform ligament, the left triangular ligament is divided (avascular plane), up to the bare area, taking care not to go too far, where the suprahepatic IVC is (danger area!).

The hepatic ligamentous attachments are divided; the falciform ligament should be already divided. Follow the falciform upwards to the IVC. Once it starts to develop into areolar tissue, stop! The hepatic veins are close by and easily torn. Develop the plane with gentle manual dissection and continue to dissect laterally to mobilise the right lobe of the liver in a medial direction.

On the left side, the left lobe is mobilised by placing a large swab behind the left triangular ligament and dividing it with electrocautery or scissors (**Figure 9.11**). The right triangular ligament is more challenging. Palpate this ligament and mobilise using tactile dissection. Be careful not to dissect too aggressively towards the midpoint of the liver, where the IVC is (danger zone). Once successfully mobilised, each liver lobe can be 'bent forwards' to open up the posterior liver for inspection. This also allows direct exposure of the retro-hepatic IVC and the major hepatic veins.

Lobar mobilisation

Lobar mobilisation is a modification of liver packing which has shown some promise in managing retro-hepatic IVC injuries. It involves mobilisation of the right lobe of the liver (as described earlier) followed by immediate packing into the para-caval, lateral and anterior aspects of the liver. Take care not to overcompress the IVC, which will reduce cardiac venous return and aggravate the shock already present. Overpacking may also lead to IVC thrombosis. As already mentioned, if there is a suspected retro-hepatic IVC injury within a *contained* retro-hepatic haematoma, then leave this undisturbed, as further mobilising of the liver may lead to rapid exsanguination.

Lobar hepatic resection

Lobar hepatic resection is rarely required in trauma and should be avoided at the index operation, as it is an injury burden on the already severely compromised patient. Mobilisation is undertaken as previously described. The relevant hepatic artery is identified and initially clamped. This allows ischaemic demarcation to occur thereby signifying the traumatised area requiring excision. If so, the respective vessel is ligated and the affected liver lobe formally resected with a mixture of finger fracture and electrocautery. Right hemi-hepatectomies are more commonly performed than left after blunt trauma, due to the large size and dominant lay of the right lobe. Resection of the right lobe of the liver can be aided by dividing the right hepatic vein prior to attempted resection.

Liver injury with massive exsanguination

If massive hepatic exsanguination is present upon opening

If there is a sense of impending doom during the trauma laparotomy and massive exsanguination seems likely, then there should be a low threshold for applying a supracoeliac aortic compression device or clamp (**Figure 9.4**) for total in-flow control. In addition, the Pringle manoeuvre should be applied immediately after hepatic packing (**Figure 9.7**). If bleeding is still not controlled, then suspect a retro-hepatic IVC injury. Further exposure will be required with or without *total vascular isolation* of the liver.

Inferior vena cava (IVC) exposure and total vascular isolation of the liver

The infra-hepatic IVC is best exposed *via* the Cattell–Braasch manoeuvre combined with a Kocher manoeuvre (see later). Total vascular isolation of the liver describes a combination of the Pringle manoeuvre (portal and arterial inflow control) combined with hepatic venous isolation (infra-hepatic IVC, supra-hepatic IVC and occasionally the hepatic veins as they arise from the posterior liver draining directly into the retro-hepatic IVC). A right subcostal incision may also aid in exposure and mobilisation of a posterior liver injury.

The supra-hepatic IVC is best exposed with a right-sided antero-lateral (or clamshell) thoracotomy (with opening of the pericardium on this side) to gain control at the level of the intra-thoracic IVC (just before it enters the right heart). This may also be combined with splitting of the diaphragm as required (split it radially and laterally through its muscular portion to avoid injuring the phrenic nerve but leaving enough cuff of diaphragmatic muscle for repair afterwards).

If a retro-hepatic IVC injury is accessible with this and rapid suturing of the injury possible, then the surgeon must work quickly to gain haemorrhage control, then re-position the liver into its bed and release any vascular liver clamping (IVC above and below and Pringle manoeuvre release). If the retro-hepatic venous injury involves disruption of the hepatic veins (these drain directly into the retro-hepatic IVC from the posterior liver) the mortality approaches 100%. However, with total hepatic isolation, the right lobe of the liver may be mobilised forwards, and the three large hepatic veins (right, left and middle) dissected and isolated as they directly enter the IVC at the back (sometimes only two are visible as the middle hepatic vein joins one or the other of the right or left hepatic veins early before exiting from the liver). Patients rarely survive this magnitude of injury as the hepatic veins are typically 'ripped off' the retro-hepatic IVC and successful repair is almost impossible. Transplantation has been reported as a salvage operation.

Atrio-caval shunting

Atrio-caval shunting is an advanced, 'last ditch' technique for managing an extensive retro-hepatic IVC injury, with no real consensus as to whether it affects mortality. After complete mobilisation of the liver and total hepatic vascular isolation, a large shunt (large plastic tube such as a 36Fr chest tube, with additional side holes cut into it with a heavy scissors to allow unrestricted through-flow) is inserted from the right heart and carefully advanced from above into the retro-hepatic IVC and into the infra-hepatic IVC for total control of the retro-hepatic venous complex (in theory). The heart is exposed either by a clamshell thoracotomy (quickest) or sternotomy and a purse string suture placed in the auricle of the right atrium. The right atrium is opened and the chest drain advanced retrograde and manually fed into the IVC below.

Ties (e.g. nylon tapes or Rummel tourniquets) are also placed around the supra-renal and infra-cardiac (supra-hepatic) IVC to hold the shunt *in situ* within the lumen of the IVC, effectively bypassing the liver and isolating the IVC. The top end of the chest tube should be clamped as it sits proud of the right heart to prevent loss of blood (blood will return to the right heart *via* the additional side holes cut in the tube). Other commercial devices are also available for the same purpose (e.g. Schrock atriocaval shunt).

Additional vascular exclusion techniques

Cardiopulmonary and veno-venous bypass have been used in massive liver trauma to allow repair of a difficult to reach liver injury or a retro-hepatic IVC injury in a bloodless field. They may also act as a bridge to transplantation with total liver destruction. In veno-venous bypass, a catheter is placed in the femoral vein and allowed to sit supra-renal/infra-hepatic, while the other catheter is placed in the right internal jugular vein and allowed to sit at the atrio-caval junction. Blood then transits *via* an extracorporeal circuit from the femoral to the jugular catheter, resulting in decreased retro-hepatic IVC blood flow. Ischaemia-reperfusion injury commonly occurs after restoration of liver perfusion.

Pancreatico-duodenal injuries

Pancreatic injuries are challenging to manage with associated high morbidity. Anatomically, the pancreas traverses the midline, within the upper retroperitoneum lying transverse across the L1 vertebral body (trans-pyloric plane), making it susceptible to crush-type injuries (e.g. Chance fracture of L1). In addition, due to its retroperitoneal position, symptoms and signs are often masked (at least initially), making early diagnosis of injury difficult (i.e. lack of peritoneal signs). A penetrating wound may be more obvious with the missile tract visible on CT. The complex vasculature surrounding the pancreas adds additional risk of massive bleeding, in particular the portal vein (confluence of the superior mesenteric and splenic veins posterior to the pancreas at the junction of the pancreatic head and tail), the inferior vena cava, the right renal pedicle, the superior mesenteric artery and the pancreatico-duodenal arcade. Haemorrhage here can be extensive and from multiple sites making it challenging to control (**Figure 9.12**).

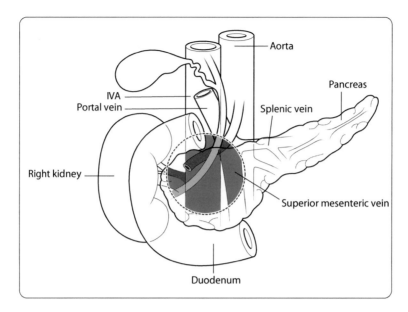

Figure 9.12 Vascular structures at risk in zone I retroperitoneal injuries. There is a dangerous conglomeration of vessels and structures in close vicinity to the pancreas and duodenum. This includes the junction of the splenic vein (retropancreatic) with the superior mesenteric vein creating the portal vein (junction of pancreatic head and tail). The portal vein then travels in the free edge of the lesser omentum. The superior mesenteric artery lies directly behind the pancreas with the coeliac complex superior, giving rise to the splenic artery (travelling along the superior border of the pancreas) and the hepatic artery (also travels in the free edge of the lesser omentum).

Additional structures in close proximity to the pancreas include: the duodenum, the spleen, the stomach, CBD and hepatic artery. Therefore, a pancreatic injury carries a high prevalence of an associated and serious concomitant injury to one or more of these structures. Management of the injured pancreas is dependent on the site of the injury relative to the superior mesenteric vessels (as they exit below the pancreas representing the demarcation of the pancreatic head from the tail). Thus, injuries are subdivided into injuries that lie either to the right hand side (pancreatic head injuries) or left hand side (pancreatic tail injuries) of the superior mesenteric vessels.

> The initial priority is haemorrhage control

Surgical exposure of the pancreas

> The pancreas has multiple surrounding vascular structures. The initial goal is haemostasis followed by full injury evaluation

A full and complete trauma laparotomy includes visualisation of the entire pancreas to rule out or define injuries, as a missed pancreatic injury carries a high morbidity. The anterior pancreas is exposed and inspected by entering the lesser sac from an anterior

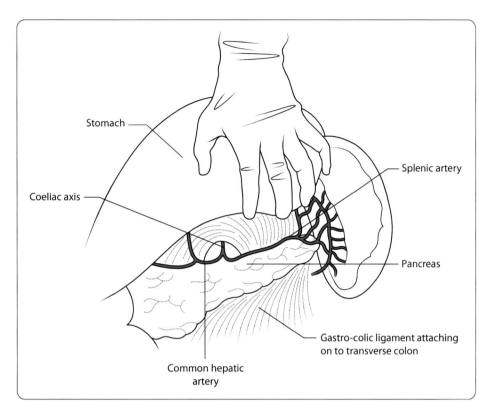

Figure 9.13 Visualisation of the pancreas. The anterior pancreas is visualised by opening the lesser sac. Stretch the stomach upwards (cephalad) and the transverse colon downwards (caudal) to stretch the gastro-colic ligament. This will be the window into the lesser sac. Ligate and divide the small vessels traversing the ligament here and open widely. This will bring the surgeon directly on to the pancreas. Note the splenic artery running along the superior border of the pancreas after exiting form the coeliac artery. The common hepatic artery is also seen traveling towards the patients right side, which in turn contributes to the pancreatic-duodenal arcade of vessels.

direct approach by elevating the stomach whilst retracting the transverse colon downwards to stretch open the gastro-colic ligament before opening it (**Figure 9.13**). This will visualise most of the anterior pancreas.

The posterior pancreas is more challenging to expose. The head of pancreas (HoP) is inspected *in unison* with the duodenum and a full *Kocher manoeuvre* (**Figures 9.14a,b** and **9.15**) is necessary (typically with a synchronous *Cattell–Braasch manoeuvre*). The peritoneal reflection lateral to D2 (relatively avascular plane) is divided (as D2 is a retroperitoneal structure) and a plane developed lateral to and behind D2 as it is reflected forwards and medially. By doing this, the posterior aspect of D2 and HoP can be inspected directly for injury. The posterior tail is best inspected by dividing the surrounding splenic ligaments (as described earlier in this chapter) and elevating the spleen with the tail of pancreas *en masse*. D4 of the duodenum is best inspected to the *left* of the superior mesenteric vessels, including division of the ligament of Treitz to allow mobilisation of the duodenojejunal (DJ) flexure.

By ritually following these manoeuvres, for every trauma laparotomy will allow for the full visualisation of the entire pancreatico-duodenal complex making a missed injury less

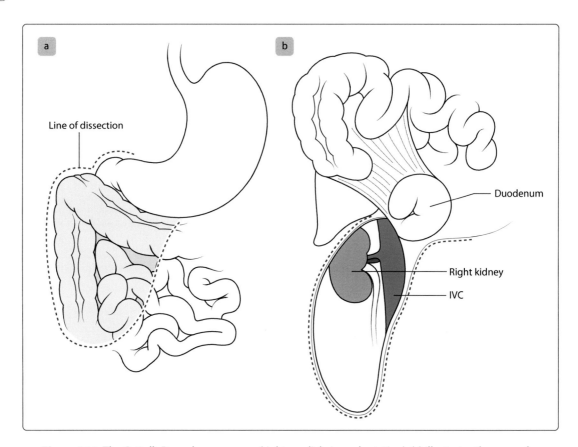

Figure 9.14 The Cattell–Braasch manoeuvre (right medial visceral rotation): (a) illustrates the avascular plane for division of the peritoneum lateral to the ascending colon (akin to the dissection for a right hemi-colectomy). (b). After division of this peritoneal 'white line' of reflection, the ascending colon and hepatic flexure are rotated upwards and medially. Continue the dissection plane to also elevate the small bowel down to the root of the mesentry and lift it out of the surgical field, thus exposing the right kidney (kept down and covered in Gerota's fascia) and IVC.

likely. As already emphasised, this area is extremely vascular, and invariably, an injury here will result in active bleeding/haematoma, in addition to spillage of pancreatic corrosive enzymatic fluid which is very pro-inflammatory.

Decision-making after pancreatic injury

Managing the injured pancreas is dependent on whether the main pancreatic duct is involved and if so, whether the injury is to the left or right of the superior mesenteric vessels

For operative management, pancreatic injuries are divided by the position of the injury relative to the *superior mesenteric vessels*. Injuries to the left (patient's left) are considered *pancreatic tail injuries* and those to the right are *HoP injuries*. In addition, *a pancreatic injury either involves the pancreatic duct or not.*

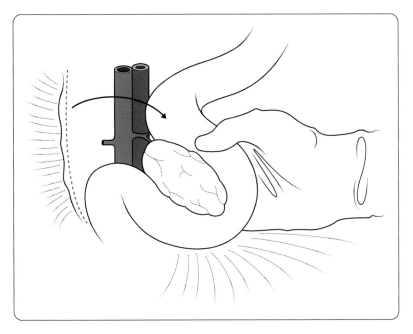

Figure 9.15 Kocher manoeuvre. The Cattell–Braasch manoeuvre described above is continued and blended with the Kocher manoeuvre. Continue the division of the lateral peritoneal reflection superior and lateral to the duodenum (D2). This allows mobilisation of the retroperitoneal duodenum forwards and medially, thus bringing the posterior aspect of both the duodenum and pancreatic head in to view (in addition to the remainder of the IVC).

No pancreatic duct injury present

These injuries may be simply debrided, irrigated and widely drained with a planned relook operation whether the tail or HoP is involved. Simple parenchymal lacerations may be repaired with a simple absorbable suture and drained.

Pancreatic duct injury present

Now the anatomical position of the injury becomes important. If the pancreatic duct injury is to the *left* of the superior mesenteric vessels, then this is a pancreatic tail injury, best managed with resection of the entire tail. This approach minimises complications that a pancreatic tail injury can bring. If the pancreatic duct injury is to the *right* of the superior mesenteric vessels, then this is a HoP injury, and a concomitant duodenal injury is highly likely. Both the HoP and duodenum share a common blood supply, so any surgical resection of the HoP will have to include the duodenum in the resection specimen (regardless of whether the duodenum is also injured or not).

Tail of pancreas resection

Typically, the spleen is included in the resection. Dissect and mobilise the spleen as described earlier (**Figure 9.5**), but elevate it farther *en masse* with the pancreatic tail (**Figure 9.16**). Develop the plane behind the tail and control the splenic vessels (the splenic artery travels along the superior border of the pancreas, giving multiple small branches to it, while the splenic vein lies posterior to the pancreas (almost within the surrounding

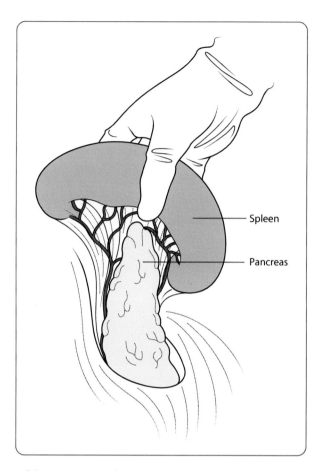

Spleen

Pancreas

Figure 9.16 Delivery of the pancreatic tail with the spleen *en masse*. If a distal pancreatectomy (tail to the left of the superior mesenteric vessels) is undertaken, elevate the spleen (dissection as described before) with the pancreatic tail *en masse* and in to the midline. Ligate the splenic artery (running along the superior border of the pancreas) and it's branches. Ligate the splenic vein (posterior pancreas) and its branches. Complete the resection by firing a GIA stapling device across the pancreas just to the left of the superior mesenteric vessels.

pancreatic tissue). Divide the pancreas approximately 1 cm from the site of injury, or if totally destroyed, just to the left of the superior mesenteric vessels (i.e. complete pancreatic tail resection). Use a linear stapler (if available) or soft bowel clamps followed by division of the tail and U-stitch. Ideally the pancreatic duct should be identified and ligated separately, but in reality, this is difficult to achieve after trauma. To reduce pancreatic leakage and fistula formation, consider adjunct techniques such as mobilising an omental pedicle and attaching it to the raw surface of the pancreas and/or applying haemostatic glue (e.g. BioGlue) to the cut surface.

If the injury is close to the neck of the pancreas (i.e. the level of the confluence of the splenic vein with the superior mesenteric vein to form the portal vein), then develop a plane anterior to the portal vein behind the pancreatic neck. Following the right gastro-epiploic vein to its confluence with the superior mesenteric vein (SMV) and the splenic vein to identify the portal vein. Insert a linear stapler arm into this space and divide. If there is limited space then

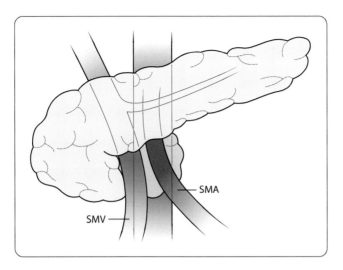

Figure 9.17 Relationship of the superior mesenteric vessels and the pancreas. The superior mesenteric artery leaves the aorta directly behind the pancreatic neck (junction of head and tail) and is best visualised as it appears just below the inferior border of the pancreas. This is the anatomical point of demarcation between the pancreatic head and tail respectively and injuries to the right or left of the vessel are managed differently.

transfix the four corners of the pancreas anterior to this plane, insert a metal spatula and divide the neck using a scalpel taking care to ligate the duct leading to the pancreatic head. The body and tail of the pancreas can then be dissected free from the splenic vein posteriorly.

Head of pancreas resection

Injuries to the HoP rarely occur in isolation and are typically high-grade, associated with a very high morbidity and mortality (**Figures 9.12**, **9.13** and **9.17**). The duodenum may be devascularised with complete destruction of the HoP and will therefore require resection of both structures (i.e. a trauma Whipple's resection), which itself is associated with a very high mortality. The best approach is to follow the damage control principles at the index operation. Debride and drain the injured HoP widely but avoid formal resection initially. Contain any duodenal contamination (**Figure 9.18**) by the various techniques described for hollow viscus injury and drain widely. Again, avoid the temptation for a formal resection at this stage, as these patients are typically very severely injured.

Once haemostasis has been achieved, stop and re-evaluate the plan of attack. You may not be able to undertake all procedures at once, thus requiring a staged approach. If a trauma Whipple's resection is required, do this as a staged procedure. At the relook operation, the duodenum (with gastric antrum) may be divided and the duodenum resected *en masse* with the HoP, by dividing the HoP to the *right* of the superior mesenteric vessels. Take care to preserve the portal vein, superior mesenteric vein, hepatic artery and CBD. The CBD may have a drain inserted directly into it, (e.g. paediatric feeding tube) and externalised for adequate drainage of the liver in the damage control setting. Do not perform the reconstruction or anastomosis until the patient is physiologically and metabolically normalised and the abdomen ready for closure, and *never reconstruct at the index operation.* Once ready for closure, the various anastomoses may be performed including pancreatico-jejunostomy, gastro-jejunostomy and choledocho-jejunostomy. This is probably best

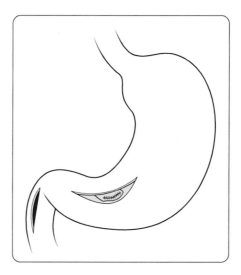

Figure 9.18 The illustration shows the pyloric exclusion technique after repair of the duodenum. A separate gastrotomy over the antrum is created and the pylorus picked up and sutured closed with either non-absorbable or absorbable (preferred) sutures to close it and protect the distal duodenal repair. This will re-open up over 7-10 days regardless due to the normal gastric and pyloric contractions.

performed at a high-volume pancreas/liver tertiary referral centre and the patient may be transferred once physiologically well enough.

If in doubt about managing such a devastating injury, then it is best to gain haemorrhage and contamination control, debride any devitalised tissue, drain widely, pack the abdomen (but leave open), and transport the patient to a pancreas/liver centre.

> Always ensure the injured pancreas is widely drained

> If a trauma Whipple's operation is required, do it as a staged procedure

Retroperitoneal injuries

> A supracoeliac clamp may be required for temporary haemorrhage control with severe retroperitoneal injuries

Severe injuries to the RP can be difficult to expose and immediately define and thus a supracoeliac clamp may be required early in the trauma laparotomy for temporary control of bleeding whilst dissection continues safely. It is not clear how long a supracoeliac clamp may remain *in situ* in severe haemorrhagic trauma, but the literature would suggest that clamp times in excess of 50–60 mins carry a 100% mortality. The retroperitoneum (RP) is divided in to three broad anatomical zones (**Figure 9.4**).

Zone I injuries

Zone I houses the major vessels in the midline (i.e. abdominal aorta, the IVC and their respective branches). All injuries here (even if only seen as a haematoma on CT or at laparotomy) must be explored as the propensity for a major exsanguinating injury is very high (regardless of the mechanism of injury). The pancreas and duodenum are also zone I structures at the superior aspect, overlying the visceral segment of the aorta (segment of the aorta where the coeliac, superior mesenteric artery and renal branches arise).

Zone II injuries

Zone II incorporates the organs and vessels in the lateral retroperitoneum (i.e. the flanks). Due to the overlying, protective Gerota's fascia in zone II, injuries here only require direct exploration after blunt trauma if there is an *expanding* or *pulsatile* haematoma (i.e. signifies arterial [high pressure] bleeding). A non-expanding or non-pulsatile haematoma has typically already self-tamponaded (as it is lower pressure venous/capillary bleeding) and may be left undisturbed. Remember, a contrast extravasation blush seen on CTA in zone II is the radiological equivalent of an arterial bleed and must also be explored. However, with penetrating injury, it is recommended to explore all zone II injuries, as the risk of a significant injury is much higher in addition to the risk of penetration of the posterior wall of the ascending or descending colon respectively (missed injury on CT), only to develop sepsis a number of days later.

Zone III injuries

Zone III is the extra-peritoneal pelvis (as discussed in Chapter 7) and contains the large iliac vessels. Similar to a zone II injury, explore the pelvis if the haematoma is pulsatile or expanding, but otherwise avoid de-roofing a stable pelvic haematoma (low pressure venous/capillary haematoma) after blunt injury. Like zone II injuries, explore all penetrating injuries to the pelvis as the prevalence of a concomitant pelvic organ injury (rectum, bladder, vagina, uterus) is much higher.

> Zone I injuries with a haematoma mandate surgical exploration regardless of mechanism of injury

Access to the retroperitoneum

As mentioned above, immediate control of major retroperitoneal bleeding may require a supracoeliac camp. The retroperitoneum may then be accessed as either:

1. Trans-peritoneal
2. Retroperitoneal
   a. Right medial visceral rotation (combined Cattell–Braasch and Kocher manoeuvres)
   b. Left medial visceral rotation (Mattox manoeuvre)

Trans-peritoneal approach

The trans-peritoneal approach allows direct access to both the anterior aorta and IVC below the level of their respective renal branches. However, although it may be the best initial approach for gross haemorrhage control, it is limited for further, more advanced exploration and is typically followed by one or both of the retroperitoneal dissection approaches described below.

Retroperitoneal approach

The retroperitoneal dissection offers the widest exposure and best approach to the RP including the vascular segments above the level of the renal vessels. A right medial visceral rotation (with or without a Kocher manoeuvre) is reserved for right-sided RP injuries (especially IVC) and a left medial visceral rotation for left-sided injuries (especially aortic). If unsure, do both!

Right medial visceral rotation

The right medial visceral rotation is also referred to as the Cattell–Braasch manoeuvre and is often combined with a Kocher manoeuvre in trauma for additional exposure. Typically, the haematoma, located to the right of the midline, is associated with a high prevalence of an IVC injury!

The peritoneal reflection (white line) at the lateral aspect of the right hemicolon (relatively avascular plane) is divided and the caecum and ascending colon mobilised towards the midline. This approach is similar to the initial dissection during a right hemicolectomy, but often, with extensive trauma or haemorrhage, the right-sided RP haematoma has done most of the dissection for the surgeon and the colon is easily mobilised forwards with little additional manual dissection. Mobilisation is continued up to include the hepatoduodenal ligament lateral to the duodenum to allow duodenal mobilisation (Kocher manoeuvre) *en masse* with the ascending colon from lateral to medial. The root of the small bowel mesentery is also mobilised *en masse* up towards the base of the superior mesenteric artery (**Figure 9.14a,b**). During Kocherisation of the duodenum (**Figure 9.15**), take care not to avulse any of the pancreatico-duodenal vessels as further significant blood loss may occur.

Once the right colon and duodenum are mobilised, this allows great exposure of the IVC from the confluence of the iliac veins up to the renal veins and higher up to the origin of the retro-hepatic IVC and porta hepatis (if required). The right kidney is typically left down in its bed during this dissection, unless it too needs to be elevated due to injury (see later). Although the likely injury will be the IVC (or its branches), once this is controlled, make sure the right ureter is directly inspected for injury (especially after penetrating trauma) so that an injury is not missed.

Injuries to the inferior vena cava

The IVC is a low-pressure (but high-flow) vessel. Therefore, *a CT scan may not reliably show evidence of injury, as the physiological compartment pressure of the abdominal cavity may tamponade haemorrhage, save for a small haematoma.* A contrast 'blush' is unlikely to be appreciated on scanning. Thus, any trauma to zone I (evidenced by the presence of a haematoma) must be explored. Always maintain a high index of suspicion for an IVC injury in this scenario.

The IVC has four anatomical segments:

1. **Infra-renal IVC** (the abdominal IVC up to the level of the renal veins and the segment most likely injured)
2. **Supra-renal IVC** (from the renal veins up to the point of where it disappears behind the liver; injuries here are often lethal)
3. **Retro-hepatic IVC** (the segment behind the liver and discussed earlier)
4. **Supra-hepatic IVC** (the segment above the liver, which in turn has two parts: The *intra-abdominal supra-hepatic IVC* and the *intra-thoracic supra-hepatic IVC*, both about 2cm long)

Once exposed, the IVC must be controlled above and below the haematoma/injury. Avoid clamping the IVC is possible, as it is a very thin-walled vessel and is unforgiving if torn. In addition, rotation of the IVC should not be attempted (will likely tear it or avulse a lumbar branch). Instead use two sponge sticks (swab-on-a-stick) to compress it above and below the injury before opening the haematoma (**Figure 9.19**). Additionally, the torn wall may be stacked with Alice clamps. Needless to say, the haematoma is the last portion to be opened.

The simplest injury is a lateral wall laceration, which may be sutured with a running non-absorbable suture (e.g. 4/0 polypropylene) or a simple interrupted repair. However, it behoves the surgeon to rule out a through-and-through injury to the IVC, as an anterior wall injury will almost always have a posterior wall injury in addition. Thus, once proximal and distal control are achieved (as described before), the anterior defect must be extended open to allow inspection of the back wall (from inside the vessel). If an injury is present on the posterior wall, this can be sutured with a running polypropylene suture (e.g. 4/0 polypropylene), leaving the surgical knots on the inside of the vessel. *Do not attempt to mobilise the IVC posteriorly.* Then, the anterior wall can be sutured in a similar manner, as previously described, before releasing the sponge-sticks.

In the unfortunate event of a catastrophic, non-reconstructable IVC injury, the DCS option is to acutely ligate the IVC (occasionally a shunt may be placed) below the level of the renal branches. Unfortunately, ligation of the suprarenal segment carries a 100% mortality. Consider performing lower limb fasciotomies after ligation due to the risk of severe lower limb swelling and potential for venous ischaemia and lower limb compartment syndrome. If fasciotomies are not performed, then ensure the limbs are dressed with compression dressings and inspected at regular intervals. In addition, the abdomen should be left open to mitigate the risk of abdominal compartment syndrome from mesenteric venous congestion and venous ischaemia of the bowel.

Left medial visceral rotation

Left medial visceral rotation is also referred to as the Mattox manoeuvre and is a mirror image dissection to its right-sided counterpart, but performed on the left colon. Typically, the haematoma is located to the left of the midline, which is associated with a high prevalence of an aortic injury. The left medial visceral rotation allows the surgeon to access the sub-diaphragmatic aorta from the its bifurcation (iliac arteries), up to the visceral aorta and its branches.

The small bowel is eviscerated to the right and the transverse colon and omentum are reflected cephalad. The left lateral peritoneal reflection (white line of Toldt) is then identified

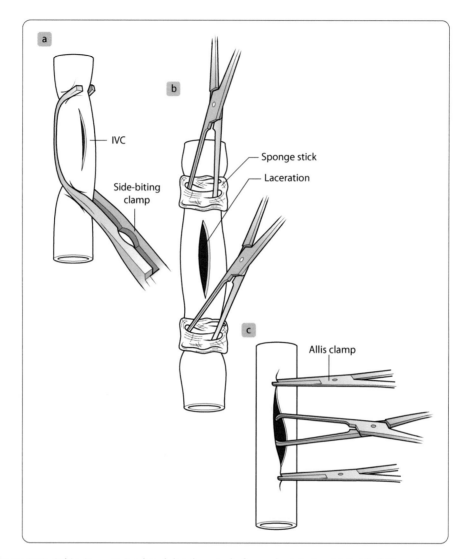

Figure 9.19 Achieving proximal and distal control of vascular injuries. (a) A side-biting clamp may be applied to the IVC at the level of the injury, but it is preferable to only compress the IVC using sponge sticks. (b) Direct pressure is applied above and below the site of injury using the sponge sticks before opening the haematoma. (c) Allis clamps may be used to pick up the torn edges of the IVC injury, however, these also carry a risk of tearing the vessel, and will not control a posterior wall injury (high likelihood with an anterior penetrating wound).

and dissected (relatively avascular plane) to allow reflection of the descending and sigmoid colons towards the midline. As with the right side, the haematoma will typically have done much of the dissection already and simple further manual dissection allows further mobilisation of the bowel and wider exposure (**Figure 9.20**).

Extend the peritoneal dissection and reflection cephalad. The left kidney may be left 'down' in its normal renal bed or elevated with the dissection *en masse*. Leaving the left kidney down is suitable for access to the infra-renal abdominal aorta, but if the visceral aorta needs inspection and repair, then the left kidney must also be elevated for

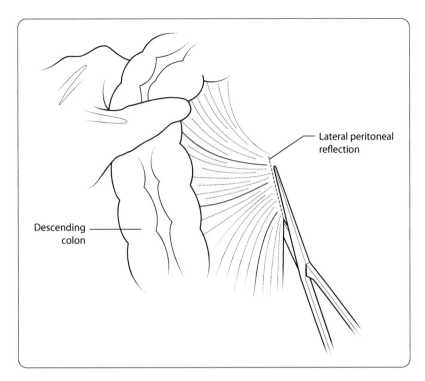

Figure 9.20 Mattox manoeuvre: Division of the peritoneum along the line of Toldt. The lateral white line of Toltz is a relatively avascular plane (often the haematoma has performed most of this dissection already). The descending colon and sigmoid are stretched towards the midline, exposing the lateral peritoneal reflection, which in turn is excised in a longitudinal fashion which allows the bowel to be mobilised further to the midline exposing the retroperitoneum.

Labels in figure: Lateral peritoneal reflection; Descending colon

exposure. Perform this by dissecting laterally along the left Gerota's fascia (very thick) and mobilising the left kidney from lateral to medial (avascular plane). Dissect posterior to the left kidney, continuing in the plane just anterior to the posterior abdominal wall musculature but posterior to the left kidney. Continue further cephalad (if you think you have gone far enough, continue until you cannot go any further) and reflect the splenic flexure of the colon and spleen with the pancreatic tail towards the midline *en masse* (**Figure 9.21**).

This gives wide exposure of the entire intra-abdominal aorta (including the visceral segment) up to the diaphragmatic hiatus. Just like its right-sided counterpart, look specifically for a left ureteric injury. This exposure allows for both proximal and distal control of the aorta (if a supracoeliac clamp had been applied, then it may now be relocated to a more appropriate position pending identification of the aortic injury).

An isolated injury to the lateral wall of the aorta may be repaired with direct suturing using a nonabsorbable suture (e.g. 3/0 polypropylene), which is the best damage control option (if the injury allows). However, more extensive injuries or large defects will require an interposition graft. This is not an ideal option in the damage control scenario due to the length of time it takes to perform in addition to the increased physiologic burden on the patient. The simplest DCS manoeuvre is to shunt the aorta (e.g. sterile, appropriately sized

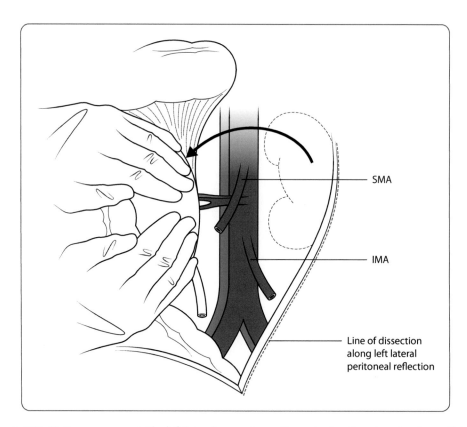

Figure 9.21 Mattox manoeuvre. The left lateral avascular peritoneal reflection plane has been divided and the left colon reflected from left to right. This lateral dissection plane is continued lateral to and behind the left kidney (and Gerota's fascia) to elevate the left kidney forward and towards the midline. Often the haematoma has performed much of the dissection already. Once performed, this allows massive exposure of the aorta from the common iliac arteries and up to the visceral aorta (i.e. segment containing the renal vessels, superior mesenteric artery and coeliac artery). Remember, the left renal artery will now be *anterior* to the aorta (and not left lateral) due to the elevation of the left kidney.

chest drain, cut to fit and held in place using nylon tapes encircling the vessel). If the patient survives, then definitive repair of the aorta may be undertaken during DCS stage III.

> The best damage control option for the aorta is to place an appropriately sized shunt

Enteric vessel injury

> You can ligate any vessel in damage control, but you must be able to deal with the consequences

If the patient is *in extremis* and actively bleeding, there may be no alternative except to tie off a bleeding vessel.

Coeliac axis

The coeliac axis may be ligated acutely, as typically there is adequate collateral supply from its natural anastomosis with branches from the superior mesenteric artery (SMA) complex (e.g. pancreatico-duodenal arcade). However, in the shocked, traumatised patient it may aggravate or lead to hepatic ischaemia.

Superior Mesenteric Artery

This should be preserved and attempts made to avoid ligating it. The incidence of total bowel necrosis is in excess of 85% with acute ligation normally, but in the shocked, traumatised patient, the overall mortality is close to 100%. Successful SMA shunting has been described and is the damage control technique of choice if a bleeding, injured SMA is encountered. This is seldom an isolated injury and likely involves additional severe injuries in close proximity, including the aorta, IVC, pancreas and duodenum.

Inferior mesenteric artery

The inferior mesenteric artery may be ligated with impunity. The incidence of acute sigmoid ischaemia is about 1% (likely higher in the shocked, traumatised patient) and thus a relook procedure is advisable in case a sigmoid colectomy is required. Therefore, leave the abdomen open!

Renal injuries

The kidneys lie in zone II (**Figures 9.2** and **9.22**) of the RP and exploration and management depends on a number of factors. After blunt trauma, a non-expanding/non-pulsatile peri-renal or zone II haematoma, may be safely left undisturbed as this typically results from a

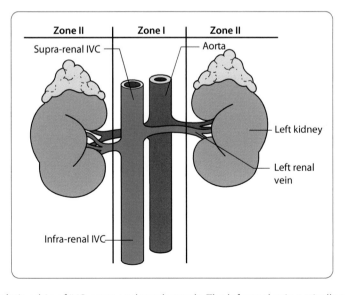

Figure 9.22 Relationship of IVC, aorta and renal vessels. The left renal vein typically travels anterior and over the aorta. However, it may be posterior (5% of population) or bifid (with anterior and posterior portions).

low-pressure (venous/capillary) bleed that will remain contained and tamponaded by the surrounding Gerota's fascia. Opening the fascia will run the unnecessary risk of further blood loss that is already safely contained. However, an expanding or pulsatile haematoma in zone II after blunt trauma signifies an arterial (high pressure) bleed which is less likely to self-tamponade with the risk of further dissection and expansion through the plane with risk of rupture (like a ruptured AAA). This must be explored and managed appropriately.

All penetrating injuries to zone II should be surgically explored, due to the high risk of arterial injury and injury to the posterior wall of the ascending and descending colon respectively. Exploration is *via* the appropriate right and left medial visceral rotation as described earlier. The kidney may be suture repaired (simple capsular lacerations) or mesh repaired (the entire kidney is wrapped in an absorbable mesh for tamponade), depending on the extent of injury. However, if there is an injury to the collecting system, this must be repaired separate to the capsular/parenchymal injury. Use absorbable suture to prevent stone formation and always drain the renal bed widely, as an urinoma is inevitable if the collecting system has been injured. For damage control with a shattered kidney, and an exsanguinating patient, a nephrectomy should be performed. Once the kidney is mobilised upwards, ligate the renal artery, renal vein and ureter separately. Trace the ureter down towards the pelvis for ligation and division if time allows to avoid leaving a redundant, atonic ureter behind (although this is not as important as historically taught).

Like in other dissections, the haematoma has often done much of the dissection through the correct plane, and the surgeon may only have to use an appropriate amount of additional blunt manual dissection to sweep the injured kidney upwards. Initially, place your hand lateral to the affected kidney (avascular plane), then scoop up the kidney, lifting it upwards by running your fingertips along the posterior abdominal musculature and into the midline. A large abdominal swab may be placed posteriorly to maintain this position. Obtain renal hilar control by squeezing the hilum between the index finger and thumb. *Note*: The right renal vein may be very short and, in some instances, absent, so in effect you will be operating upon the IVC.

> There is no role for renal conservation in the physiologically compromised exsanguinating patient

Absence of a kidney on the other side will not make the patient's physiology better and, more important, should not influence the procedure. The goal is to achieve a live patient!

Ureteric injuries

Ureteric injuries should be suspected in all penetrating zone I and II injuries. The key to management is awareness and early identification of the intact ureter (and noted in the post-op note). Make sure you specifically inspect for the ureter. In the DCS scenario, a ureteric injury is best managed by placing a draining tube (e.g. small feeding tube) and externalising it through the skin. In addition, also place a drain adjacent to the injured organ. Only undertake definitive ureteric repairs if you have the necessary skill set, as these injuries are not life threatening and can wait for urology consultation. If a repair is undertaken, spatulate the ends of the ureter for direct anastomosis (to prevent stenosis) and use an interrupted absorbable suture (to prevent stone formation) and repair over a double-J stent placed caudal (into the bladder) and cephalad (into the renal hilar collecting system) and palpated manually for position. This will be removed later by urology and after healing of the ureter.

Bladder injuries

Bladder injuries will bleed, as its musculature has a rich blood supply, but bleeding is not typically catastrophic and may just present with gross haematuria and pain. Injuries may be blunt or penetrating trauma and a bladder injury must always be suspected with pelvic fractures, especially 'open book' fractures.

A bladder rupture may be *intraperitoneal* or *extraperitoneal*. Intraperitoneal ruptures may present with signs of peritonitis (typically absent or delayed), whereas an extraperitoneal rupture may have limited signs (save for soft tissue and bony signs if a pelvic fracture is present). A high index of suspicion is indicated! Blood at the urethral meatus may be an indicator of bladder/lower urinary tract injury (or even urethral tear), but is not always present.

An extraperitoneal injury is best diagnosed with a retrograde cystogram (in the trauma bay) or a micturating CT urogram and is managed non-operatively with urinary catheter drainage for up to 2 weeks. An intraperitoneal rupture however requires operative repair, performed in two layers using absorbable suture (to avoid stone formation) with urinary catheter drainage (reduce bladder tone and contraction) and a large pelvic drain (to drain the expected urinoma). If the patient is physiologically compromised, do not repair at the index operation. Instead, place a urinary catheter (suprapubic if necessary) and a large pelvic drain for damage control and undertake repair when physiologically well enough.

Hollow viscus injuries

The hollow viscus organs include; the stomach (including the gastro-oesophageal junction), duodenum (mostly retroperitoneal), small bowel, colon (of which the ascending and descending portions are retroperitoneal) and the rectum (mostly extraperitoneal in zone III of the pelvis). Typically, the management of hollow viscus injury and control of contamination takes place *after* haemorrhage control, as these injuries are not typically as time critical (keeping in mind that they may bleed however and thus managing bleeding may also correspond with containing the contamination). The most common hollow viscus injury (blunt and penetrating) is the small bowel, which is also the most likely source of hollow viscus bleeding (rich arcade of vessels in the mesentry).

Small bowel injuries

Small bowel injuries are relatively straightforward to manage but are often multiple. The entire bowel (from DJ flexure to terminal ileum) must be inspected (front and back, mesenteric and anti-mesenteric borders). The aim of damage control is to control and contain contamination. *Primary repair and anastomosis must not be attempted in the physiologically compromised patient.* Any attempt at repair or reconstruction or anastomosis is unnecessary and dangerous in DCS, as it takes too long to complete (adding to the physiologic burden with propensity to aggravate bleeding) and the anastomosis is highly likely to fail and leak anyway, due to the shocked tissues. Control of perforated bowel

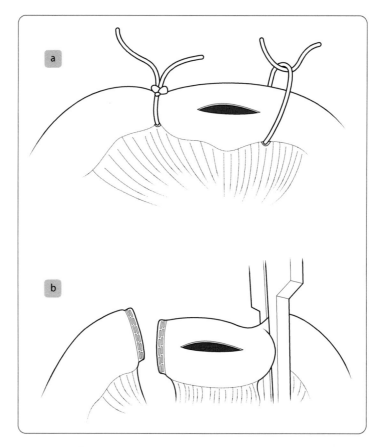

Figure 9.23 Bowel injury damage control: (a) Tying off bowel ends with nylon tape.
(b) Linear staple use.

may be obtained by a variety of methods including rapid firing of linear staplers, tying off bowel ends with nylon tape, and rapid whip suturing (or surgical clipping) of perforations (**Figure 9.23a,b**).

If extensive destruction of a segment of bowel is present, then a rapid resection of the injured piece may be necessary using linear staplers, with rapid ligation of the mesenteric blood supply. Then, leave the stapled ends of small bowel in discontinuity and delay the reconstruction until DCS stage III. An ileus is highly likely anyway and the risk of a blind loop of bowel perforating is very small. Rapidly wash out any gross contamination before applying temporary abdominal closure.

Gastric injuries

Significant gastric tissue loss is unusual after blunt trauma, as it has an excellent blood supply (thus may bleed heavily if injured). The surgeon should remain vigilant for injuries at certain key areas:

- Gastro-oesophageal junction (GOJ)
- Origin of the short gastric arteries
- Peri-pyloric region

In penetrating trauma, the degree of tissue loss depends on mechanism of penetration, that is, stab wounds create low energy wounds compared with the higher energy dump with ballistic trauma.

As with small bowel injuries, the key is contamination control. However, due to its excellent blood supply, simple lacerations may be repaired primarily. Be sure to inspect both the anterior and posterior walls of the stomach to avoid a missed injury that will later leak. This may include extending an anterior wound and inspecting the posterior wall of the stomach for injury from the inside. Always make a point of visualising and palpating the GOJ (notorious as a site of missed injury).

More significant tissue loss and contamination may be managed with linear staplers or a running suture. We advocate nasogastric (NG) drainage of the stomach to manage secretions in addition to a post-pyloric feeding tube if a delay in feeding is predicted. Take care not to incorporate the NG tube in the linear staple/suture! If the suture is simply a damage control suture, then definitive repair may be undertaken at the relook laparotomy, especially if a more extensive reconstruction is necessary (e.g. gastrojejunostomy), but do not perform an extensive reconstruction or complex drainage procedure at the index operation.

Duodenal injuries

Duodenal injuries are discussed earlier with pancreatic injuries due to their close association shared blood supply and prevalance of dual injury.

Colonic injuries

The most common site of injury or 'missed' injury is the transverse colon (a missed injury may be obscured by the overlying thick greater omentum or a low-lying greater curve of stomach). If DCS is indicated, then rapid suturing is probably best. Most definitive repairs of a large bowel injury can also be managed with primary repair and a covering stoma is typically unnecessary, despite historical claims to the contrary, as long as the blood supply is not compromised. If the ascending or descending colon require mobilising, this is performed as the Cattell–Braasch and Mattox manoeuvres respectively. Injuries here are likely to have additional RP zone II injuries. Mobilise the left side down as far as the peritoneal reflection of the rectum. As with the small bowel, the colon may be left in discontinuity in the setting of DCS for up to 36–48 hours.

An intraperitoneal rectal injury may be managed in the same way as colonic if small but more extensive injuries will likely require externalisation of an end colostomy with delayed reconstruction. Extraperitoneal rectal injuries may be managed with a proximal diverting stoma only and without formal exposure of the extraperitoneal rectum itself. Occasionally washout and drainage of the extraperitoneal pelvis is required if heavily contaminated.

Diaphragmatic injuries

Diaphragmatic injuries are commonly missed as there is no one reliable, non-invasive diagnostic investigation to rule these in or out. In blunt trauma, they are more common on the left compared with the right (the liver offers protection on the right). In penetrating trauma, both sides are equally susceptible to injury. The diaphragmatic domes reach as far as the level of the nipples (T4) during expiration, therefore any penetrating injury to the thoracic

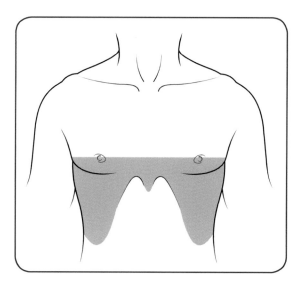

Figure 9.24 The thoraco-abdominal junctional zone: This zone of potential diaphragmatic injury stretches from the level of the nipples down to the costal margins. Any penetrating injury within this zone carries a higher prevalence of diaphragmatic injury and it behoves the surgeon to rule this out!

cavity at or below this level mandates exclusion of a diaphragmatic injury (**Figure 9.24**). We would advocate using diagnostic laparoscopy in the haemodynamically well patient to rule out a diaphragmatic injury (and obviously a laparotomy if haemodynamically unwell). Laparoscopy offers excellent visualisation of the left hemi diaphragm and LUQ (to rule out associated injury) and, if the skill set allows, laparoscopic repair (if no other injuries demand open exploration). During open surgery, diaphragmatic injury is best examined by direct palpation. If a defect is palpated, then additional exposure and visualisation will be required before undertaking a repair.

Diaphragmatic Repair

The diaphragm may be repaired from either within the chest (if a thoracotomy is already taking place) or from within the abdomen. Preferentially, repair should be *via* laparotomy, as the prevalence of a concomitant intra-abdominal injury requiring surgical management is much greater compared with the need for direct surgical management of a concomitant intra-thoracic injury. We advocate repairing the diaphragm using a full thickness, two-layer, non-absorbable heavy suture (e.g. 2/0 nylon or polypropylene). The suture may be intermittent or continuous, and may be reinforced with a Teflon buttress. Ensure the ends of the suture do not protrude against any viscus (including the heart) where erosion and perforation may occur over time with the life-long diaphragmatic movement of respiration. Occasionally, with extensive destruction, a non-absorbable mesh repair is necessary. In addition, avoid damaging the phrenic nerve endings on the thoracic side of the diaphragmatic dome.

Additional reading

Andeweg CS, Vingerhoedt NM, van Vugt AB, Haerkens MH. [Damage control surgery in polytraumatized patients]. *Ned Tijdschr Geneeskd* 2006;150(27):1503–15037.

Arhinful E, Jenkins D, Schiller HJ, Cullinane DC, Smoot DL, Zielinski MD. Outcomes of damage control laparotomy with open abdomen management in the octogenarian population. *J Trauma* 2011;70(3):616–621.

Arul GS, Sonka BJ, Lundy JB, Rickard RF, Jeffery SL. Management of complex abdominal wall defects associated with penetrating abdominal trauma. *J R Army Med Corps* 2015;161(1):46–52.

Asensio JA, Petrone P, Roldan G, Kuncir E, Ramicone E, Chan L. Has evolution in awareness of guidelines for institution of damage control improved outcome in the management of the posttraumatic open abdomen? *Arch Surg* 2004;139(2):209–214; discussion 215.

Baghdanian AA, Baghdanian AH, Khalid M et al. Damage control surgery: Use of diagnostic CT after life-saving laparotomy. *Emerg Radiol* 2016;23(5):483–495.

Ball CG. Damage control surgery. *Curr Opin Crit Care*, 2015;21(6):538–543.

Bansal V, Coimbra R. Nutritional support in patients following damage control laparotomy with an open abdomen. *Eur J Trauma Emerg Surg* 2013;39(3):243–248.

Bashir MM, Abu-Zidan FM. Damage control surgery for abdominal trauma. *Eur J Surg Suppl* 2003;(588):8–13.

Beuran M, Iordache FM. Damage control surgery—New concept or reenacting of a classical idea? *J Med Life*, 2008;1(3):247–253.

Biondo S. [Damage control surgery in non-traumatic abdominal emergencies]. *Cir Esp* 2012;90(6):345–347.

Boel T, Hillingso JG, Svendsen LB. [Damage control surgery—A survey of a Cochrane review]. *Ugeskr Laeger* 2011;173(18):1291–1293.

Bograd B, Rodriguez C, Amdur R, Gage F, Elster E, Dunne J. Use of damage control and the open abdomen in combat. *Am Surg*, 2013;79(8):747–753.

Bradley MJ, Dubose JJ, Scalea TM et al. Independent predictors of enteric fistula and abdominal sepsis after damage control laparotomy: Results from the prospective AAST Open Abdomen registry. *JAMA Surg* 2013;148(10):947–954.

Brasel KJ, Weigelt JA. Damage control in trauma surgery. *Curr Opin Crit Care* 2000;6(4):276–280.

Breeze J, Lewis EA, Fryer R, Hepper AE, Mahoney PF, Clasper JC. Defining the essential anatomical coverage provided by military body armour against high energy projectiles. *J R Army Med Corps* 2016;162(4):284–290.

Briusov PG. [Multistage surgery tactics ("damage control") in the treatment of patients with multiple trauma]. *Voen Med Zh* 2008;329(4):19–24.

Chaudhry R, Tiwari GL, Singh Y. Damage control surgery for abdominal trauma. *Med J Armed Forces India*, 2006;62(3):259–262.

Choi SB, You J, Choi SY. A case of traumatic pancreaticoduodenal injury: A simple and an organ-preserving approach as damage control surgery. *JOP* 2012;13(1):76–79.

Cirocchi R, Abraha I, Montedori A et al. Damage control surgery for abdominal trauma. *Cochrane Database Syst Rev* 2010(1):CD007438.

Cirocchi R, Montedori A, Farinella E, Bonacini I, Tagliabue L, Abraha I. Damage control surgery for abdominal trauma. *Cochrane Database Syst Rev* 2013;(3):CD007438.

Diaz JJ Jr., Cullinane DC, Dutton WD et al. The management of the open abdomen in trauma and emergency general surgery: Part 1 – Damage control. *J Trauma* 2010;68(6):1425–1438.

Dubose JJ, Scalea TM, Holcomb JB et al. Open abdominal management after damage-control laparotomy for trauma: A prospective observational American Association for the Surgery of Trauma multicenter study. *J Trauma Acute Care Surg* 2013;74(1):113–120; discussion 1120–1122.

Ebihara T, Yamada M, Simizu K et al. [Damage control surgery for perforation of colon cancer]. *Gan To Kagaku Ryoho* 2016;43(12):1830–1832.

Edelmuth RC, Buscariolli Ydos S, Ribeiro MA Jr. [Damage control surgery: An update]. *Rev Col Bras Cir*, 2013;40(2):142–151.

Eiseman B, Moore EE, Meldrum DR, Raeburn C. Feasibility of damage control surgery in the management of military combat casualties. *Arch Surg* 2000;135(11):1323–1327.

Ewertsen C, Hansen KL, Nielsen MB. [Aspects of imaging modalities in relation to damage control surgery]. *Ugeskr Laeger* 2011;173(18):1267–1270.

Ferguson EJ, Oswanski MF, Stombaugh HA, Daniels RG. Early definitive closure of abdomen using components separation technique after damage control surgery. *Am Surg* 2011;77(4):E74–E75.

Finlay IG, Edwards TJ, Lambert AW. Damage control laparotomy. *Br J Surg* 2004;91(1):83–85.

Fox N, Crutchfield M, LaChant M, Ross SE, Seamon MJ. Early abdominal closure improves long-term outcomes after damage-control laparotomy. *J Trauma Acute Care Surg* 2013;75(5):854–858.

Fries CA, Penn-Barwell J, Tai NR, Hodgetts TJ, Midwinter MJ, Bowley DM. Management of intestinal injury in deployed UK hospitals. *J R Army Med Corps* 2011;157(4):370–373.

Germanos S, Gourgiotis S, Villias C, Bertucci M, Dimopoulos N, Salemis N. Damage control surgery in the abdomen: An approach for the management of severe injured patients. *Int J Surg* 2008;6(3):246–252.

Glasgow SC, Steele SR, Duncan JE, Rasmussen TE. Epidemiology of modern battlefield colorectal trauma: A review of 977 coalition casualties. *J Trauma Acute Care Surg*, 2012;73(6 Suppl 5):S503–S508.

Godat L, Kobayashi L, Costantini T, Coimbra R. Abdominal damage control surgery and reconstruction: World society of emergency surgery position paper. *World J Emerg Surg* 2013;8(1):53.

Goldberg SR, Henning J, Wolfe LG, Duane TM. Practice patterns for the use of antibiotic agents in damage control laparotomy and its impact on outcomes. *Surg Infect (Larchmt)* 2017;18(3):282–286.

Goncalves R, Saad R Jr. Thoracic damage control surgery. *Rev Col Bras Cir* 2016;43(5):374–381.

Griggs C, Butler K. Damage control and the open abdomen: Challenges for the nonsurgical intensivist. *J Intensive Care Med* 2016;31(9):567–576.

Ham AA, Coveler LA. Anesthetic considerations in damage control surgery. *Surg Clin North Am*, 1997;77(4):909–920.

Hamill J. Damage control surgery in children. *Injury* 2004;35(7):708–712.

Haricharan RN, Dooley AC, Weinberg JA et al. Body mass index affects time to definitive closure after damage control surgery. *J Trauma* 2009;66(6):1683–1687.

Hillingso JG, Svendsen LB, Johansson PI. [Resuscitation and abdominal surgical aspects of damage control surgery]. *Ugeskr Laeger* 2011;173(18):1271–1273.

Hirshberg A, Walden R. Damage control for abdominal trauma. *Surg Clin North Am* 1997;77(4):813–820.

Hoey BA, Schwab CW. Damage control surgery. *Scand J Surg* 2002;91(1):92–103.

Hommes M, Chowdhury S, Visconti D et al. Contemporary damage control surgery outcomes: 80 patients with severe abdominal injuries in the right upper quadrant analyzed. *Eur J Trauma Emerg Surg* 2018;44(1):79–85.

Hommes M, Kazemier G, Schep NW, Kuipers EJ, Schipper IB. Management of biliary complications following damage control surgery for liver trauma. *Eur J Trauma Emerg Surg* 2013;39(5):511–516.

Ikegami K. [Damage control surgery]. *Nihon Geka Gakkai Zasshi* 1999;100(7):430–434.

Ji W, Ding W, Liu X et al. Intraintestinal drainage as a damage control surgery adjunct in a hypothermic traumatic shock swine model with multiple bowel perforations. *J Surg Res* 2014;192(1):170–176.

Kapan M, Onder A, Oguz A et al. The effective risk factors on mortality in patients undergoing damage control surgery. *Eur Rev Med Pharmacol Sci* 2013;17(12):1681–1687.

Karamarkovic AR, Popovic NM, Blagojevic ZB et al. [Damage control surgery in abdominal trauma]. *Acta Chir Iugosl* 2010;57(1):15–24.

Kataoka Y, Minehara H, Kashimi F et al. Hybrid treatment combining emergency surgery and intraoperative interventional radiology for severe trauma. *Injury* 2016;47(1):59–63.

Khan A, Hsee L, Mathur S, Civil I. Damage-control laparotomy in nontrauma patients: Review of indications and outcomes. *J Trauma Acute Care Surg* 2013;75(3):365–368.

Khan M. Abdominal trauma. In Porter K, Greaves I, Burke D, eds. *Key Clinical Topics in Trauma*. London: JP Medical Publishers, 2016: 1–5.

Khan, M. Entero-atmospheric fistula. In Papadakos PJ, Gestring ML, eds. *Encyclopedia of Trauma Care*. Berlin: Springer, 2015: 543–544.

Khan, M. *Gastric injury*. In Papadakos PJ, Gestring ML, eds. *Encyclopedia of Trauma Care*. Berlin: Springer, 2015:146–152.

Khan, M. Gastric necrosis from short gastric embolization. In Papadakos PJ, Gestring ML, eds. *Encyclopedia of Trauma Care*. Berlin: Springer, 2015: 673–674.

Khan, M. Gastrocutaneous fistula. In Papadakos PJ, Gestring ML, eds. *Encyclopedia of Trauma Care*. Berlin: Springer, 2015: 676–677.

Khan, M. Hemobilia. In Papadakos PJ, Gestring ML, eds. *Encyclopedia of Trauma Care*. Berlin: Springer, 2015: 717–718.

Khan, M. Prolonged open abdomen. In Papadakos PJ, Gestring ML, eds. *Encyclopedia of Trauma Care*. Berlin: Springer, 2015: 1355–1356.

Khan M, Garner J. Abdominal trauma. In *Oxford Desk Reference: Major Trauma*. Oxford: Oxford University Press, 2011: 209–236.

Kirkpatrick AW, LaPorta A, Brien S et al. Technical innovations that may facilitate real-time telementoring of damage control surgery in austere environments: A proof of concept comparative evaluation of the importance of surgical experience, telepresence, gravity and mentoring in the conduct of damage control laparotomies. *Can J Surg* 2015;58(3 Suppl 3):S88–S90.

Kobayashi K. [Damage control surgery – A historical view]. *Nihon Geka Gakkai Zasshi* 2002;103(7):500–502.

Kossmann T, Trease L, Freedman I, Malham G. Damage control surgery for spine trauma. *Injury* 2004;35(7):661–670.

Kouraklis G, Spirakos S, Glinavou A. Damage control surgery: An alternative approach for the management of critically injured patients. *Surg Today* 2002;32(3):195–202.

Kushimoto S, Miyauchi M, Yokota H, Kawai M. Damage control surgery and open abdominal management: Recent advances and our approach. *J Nippon Med Sch* 2009;76(6):280–290.

Lamb CM, MacGoey P, Navarro AP, Brooks AJ. Damage control surgery in the era of damage control resuscitation. *Br J Anaesth* 2014;113(2):242–249.

Lausevic ZD, Resanovic VR, Vukovic GM et al. [Damage control surgery – Our experience]. *Acta Chir Iugosl* 2010;57(4):69–73.

Lee KJ, Kwon J, Kim J, Jung K. Management of blunt pancreatic injury by applying the principles of damage control surgery: Experience at a single institution. *Hepatogastroenterology* 2012;59(118):1970–1975.

Leppaniemi AK, Mentula PJ, Streng MH, Koivikko MP, Handolin LE. Severe hepatic trauma: Nonoperative management, definitive repair, or damage control surgery? *World J Surg* 2011;35(12):2643–2649.

Liu QW, Zhou BJ, Qin HX, Sun K. [Application of damage control surgery for severe abdominal trauma]. *Zhonghua Wei Chang Wai Ke Za Zhi* 2011;14(7):506–508.

Mani NB, Kim L. The role of interventional radiology in urologic tract trauma. *Semin Intervent Radiol* 2011;28(4):415–423.

Manterola C, Flores P, Otzen T. Floating stoma: An alternative strategy in the context of damage control surgery. *J Visc Surg* 2016;153(6):419–424.

Matsumoto H, Mashiko K, Sakamoto Y, Kutsukata N, Hara Y, Yokota H. A new look at criteria for damage control surgery. *J Nippon Med Sch* 2010;77(1):13–20.

Miller RS, Morris JA Jr., Diaz JJ Jr., Herring MB, May AK. Complications after 344 damage-control open celiotomies. *J Trauma* 2005;59(6):1365–1371; discussion 1371–1374.

Moore EE, Burch JM, Franciose RJ, Offner PJ, Biffl WL. Staged physiologic restoration and damage control surgery. *World J Surg* 1998;22(12):1184–1190; discussion 1190–1191.

Morgan K, Mansker D, Adams DB. Not just for trauma patients: Damage control laparotomy in pancreatic surgery. *J Gastrointest Surg* 2010;14(5):768–772.

Moriwaki Y, Kato M, Toyoda H et al. [Experience of damage control as the primary surgery for thoraco-abdominal injury with hemorrhagic shock]. *Kyobu Geka* 2010;63(2):112–115.

Morrison JJ. Noncompressible torso hemorrhage. *Crit Care Clin* 2017;33(1):37–54.

Mutafchiiski V, Popivanov G. Damage control surgery and open abdomen in trauma patients with exsanguinating bleeding. *Khirurgiia (Sofiia)* 2014;(1):4–10.

O'Connor JV, DuBose JJ, Scalea TM. Damage-control thoracic surgery: Management and outcomes. *J Trauma Acute Care Surg* 2014;77(5):660–665.

Pape HC, Hildebrand F, Pertschy S et al. Changes in the management of femoral shaft fractures in polytrauma patients: From early total care to damage control orthopedic surgery. *J Trauma* 2002;53(3):452–461; discussion 461–462.

Park CY, Ju JK, Kim JC. Damage control surgery in patient with delayed rupture of pseudoaneurysm after blunt abdominal trauma. *J Korean Surg Soc* 2012;83(2):119–122.

Parker PJ. Damage control surgery and casualty evacuation: Techniques for surgeons, lessons for military medical planners. *J R Army Med Corps* 2006;152(4):202–211.

Penninga L, Penninga EI, Svendsen LB. [Damage control surgery in multiply traumatised patients]. *Ugeskr Laeger* 2005;167(36):3403–3407.

Prichayudh S, Sirinawin C, Sriussadaporn S et al. Management of liver injuries: Predictors for the need of operation and damage control surgery. *Injury* 2014;45(9):1373–1377.

Raeburn CD, Moore EE, Biffl WL et al. The abdominal compartment syndrome is a morbid complication of postinjury damage control surgery. *Am J Surg* 2001;182(6):542–546.

Rago A, Duggan MJ, Marini J et al. Self-expanding foam improves survival following a lethal, exsanguinating iliac artery injury. *J Trauma Acute Care Surg* 2014;77(1):73–77.

Ribeiro MA Jr., Barros EA, de Carvalho SM, Nascimento VP, Cruvinel Neto J, Fonseca AZ. Open abdomen in gastrointestinal surgery: Which technique is the best for temporary closure during damage control? *World J Gastrointest Surg* 2016;8(8):590–597.

Roberts DJ, Bobrovitz N, Zygun DA et al. Indications for use of damage control surgery in civilian trauma patients: A content analysis and expert appropriateness rating study. *Ann Surg* 2016;263(5):1018–1027.

Roberts DJ, Bobrovitz N, Zygun DA et al. Indications for use of damage control surgery and damage control interventions in civilian trauma patients: A scoping review. *J Trauma Acute Care Surg* 2015;78(6):1187–1196.

Rotondo MF, Schwab CW, McGonigal MD et al. 'Damage control': An approach for improved survival in exsanguinating penetrating abdominal injury. *J Trauma* 1993;35(3):375–382; discussion 382–383.

Sagraves SG, Toschlog EA, Rotondo MF. Damage control surgery – The intensivist's role. *J Intensive Care Med* 2006;21(1):5–16.

Sambasivan CN, Underwood SJ, Cho SD et al. Comparison of abdominal damage control surgery in combat versus civilian trauma. *J Trauma* 2010;69(Suppl 1):S168–S174.

Shah SM, Shah KS, Joshi PK, Somani RB, Gohil VB, Dakhda SM. To study the incidence of organ damage and post-operative care in patients of blunt abdominal trauma with haemoperitoneum managed by laparoscopy. *J Minim Access Surg* 2011;7(3):169–172.

Sharrock AE, Barker T, Yuen HM, Rickard R, Tai N. Management and closure of the open abdomen after damage control laparotomy for trauma: A systematic review and meta-analysis. *Injury* 2016;47(2):296–306.

Shen XJ, Xue XC, Wang Y et al. [Predictors of mortality in critically multiple trauma patients after damage control surgery]. *Zhonghua Wai Ke Za Zhi* 2009;47(10):755–757.

Smith BP, Adams RC, Doraiswamy VA et al. Review of abdominal damage control and open abdomens: Focus on gastrointestinal complications. *J Gastrointestin Liver Dis* 2010;19(4):425–435.

Smith IM, Beech ZK, Lundy JB, Bowley DM. A prospective observational study of abdominal injury management in contemporary military operations: Damage control laparotomy is associated with high survivability and low rates of fecal diversion. *Ann Surg* 2015;261(4):765–773.

Smith JW, Garrison RN, Matheson PJ, Franklin GA, Harbrecht BG, Richardson JD. Direct peritoneal resuscitation accelerates primary abdominal wall closure after damage control surgery. *J Am Coll Surg* 2010;210(5):658–664, 664–667.

Smith JW, Matheson PJ, Franklin GA, Harbrecht BG, Richardson JD, Garrison RN. Randomized controlled trial evaluating the efficacy of peritoneal resuscitation in the management of trauma patients undergoing damage control surgery. *J Am Coll Surg* 2017;224(4):396–404.

Smith JW, Nash N, Procter L et al. Not all abdomens are the same: A comparison of damage control surgery for intra-abdominal sepsis versus trauma. *Am Surg* 2016;82(5):427–432.

Sorrentino TA, Moore EE, Wohlauer MV et al. Effect of damage control surgery on major abdominal vascular trauma. *J Surg Res* 2012;177(2):320–325.

Stagnitti F, Mongardini M, Schillaci F et al. [Damage control surgery: The technique]. *G Chir* 2002;23(1–2):18–21.

Stawicki SP, Brooks A, Bilski T et al. The concept of damage control: Extending the paradigm to emergency general surgery. *Injury* 2008;39(1):93–101.

Subramanian A, Balentine C, Palacio CH, Sansgiry S, Berger DH, Awad SS. Outcomes of damage-control celiotomy in elderly nontrauma patients with intra-abdominal catastrophes. *Am J Surg* 2010;200(6):783–788; discussion 788–789.

Sugrue M, D'Amours SK, Joshipura M. Damage control surgery and the abdomen. *Injury* 2004;35(7):642–648.

Sutton E, Bochicchio GV, Bochicchio K et al. Long term impact of damage control surgery: A preliminary prospective study. *J Trauma* 2006;61(4):831–834; discussion 835–836.

Tai N, Parker P. The damage control surgery set: Rethinking for contingency. *J R Army Med Corps* 2013;159(4):314–315.

Timmermans J, Nicol A, Kairinos N, Teijink J, Prins M, Navsaria P. Predicting mortality in damage control surgery for major abdominal trauma. *S Afr J Surg* 2010;48(1):6–9.

Tong DC, Breeze J. Damage control surgery and combat-related maxillofacial and cervical injuries: A systematic review. *Br J Oral Maxillofac Surg* 2016;54(1):8–12.

Tugnoli G, Casali M, Villani S, Biscardi A, Sinibaldi G, Baldoni F. [The damage control surgery]. *Ann Ital Chir* 2007;78(2):81–84.

Wang P, Wei X, Li Y, Li J. Influences of intestinal ligation on bacterial translocation and inflammatory response in rats with hemorrhagic shock: Implications for damage control surgery. *J Invest Surg* 2008;21(5):244–254.

Weber DG, Bendinelli C, Balogh ZJ. Damage control surgery for abdominal emergencies. *Br J Surg* 2014;101(1):e109–e118.

Xian-kai H, Yu-jun Z, Lian-yang Z. Damage control surgery for severe thoracic and abdominal injuries. *Chin J Traumatol* 2007;10(5):279–283.

Ye Z, Yang Y, Luo G, Huang Y. [Management of colonic injuries in the setting of damage control surgery]. *Zhonghua Wei Chang Wai Ke Za Zhi* 2014;17(11):1125–1129.

Yokota J. [Paradigm shift from standard surgery to damage control surgery in major trauma]. *Nihon Geka Gakkai Zasshi* 2002;103(7):503–506.

Yukioka T, Muraoka A, Kanai N. [Abdominal compartment syndrome following damage-control surgery: Pathophysiology and decompression of intraabdominal pressure]. *Nihon Geka Gakkai Zasshi* 2002;103(7):529–535.

Zhao ZG, Li YS, Wang J et al. [Damage control surgery for pancreatic injuries after blunt abdominal trauma]. *Zhonghua Wai Ke Za Zhi* 2012;50(4):299–301.

10 Future of Trauma Surgery: Resuscitative Endovascular Balloon Occlusion of the Aorta (REBOA)

Philip J. Wasicek, Thomas M. Scalea and Jonathan J. Morrison

Introduction

Haemorrhage constitutes the leading cause of preventable or reversible death and disability after major trauma. Death from major haemorrhage is theoretically preventable with prompt control of the major compelling source of bleeding followed by appropriate and targeted resuscitation. Torso haemorrhage is particularly challenging to control, as the source is within a non-compressible cavity, leading to difficulty with early identification in addition to challenging rapid surgical access.

The mortality from major torso haemorrhage remains high, with a recent U.S. National Trauma Databank analysis demonstrating a death rate approaching 40%. Similar rates have also been reported in Europe and the UK Trauma Audit and Research Network (TARN) analysis with mortalities of up to 30%. Furthermore, the injury burden, pre-hospital time and time to intervention, all rate-limiting factors in haemorrhage control, have been demonstrated as directly affecting outcomes. Even in high-volume trauma systems, the delivery of critical patients from the scene to definitive surgical haemostasis takes time and a proportion of patients exsanguinate even prior to attempted intervention.

Severe torso haemorrhage requires urgent access for haemostasis, which historically is *via* operative (open surgical) control (e.g. thoracotomy, laparotomy); however, endovascular techniques are being increasingly utilised (e.g. embolisation, stent graft insertion) with reported good success.

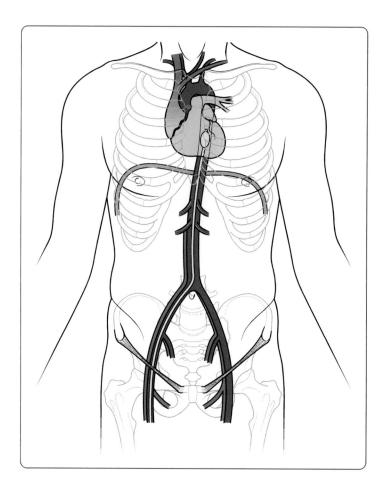

Figure 10.1 Inflation of balloon catheter in the thoracic zone (Zone 1) to achieve abdominal inflow control. The REBOA balloon is introduced *via* the femoral vessel in the groin and passed into the aorta, advancing up to the descending thoracic aorta.

Resuscitative endovascular balloon occlusion of the aorta (REBOA) is one of a growing number of *torso haemorrhage adjuncts* that have been developed in recent years and is currently undergoing further clinical evaluation. It is a haemorrhage control technique and resuscitation adjunct, designed for timely access to support the circulation prior to more definitive haemostasis. REBOA consists of a compliant balloon catheter, inserted *via* the femoral artery, navigated into the aorta and inflated in either its thoracic (zone 1) or infra-renal (zone 3) zones to achieve abdominal and/or pelvic inflow control (**Figures 10.1** and **10.2**).

This chapter aims to introduce the theory, practical steps and current evidence around the use of REBOA, while also touching on potential other future developments.

Physiology of aortic occlusion in trauma

Occluding the aorta results in profound haemodynamic alterations that can lead to significant end-organ effects, both distal and proximal to the level of the occluding balloon.

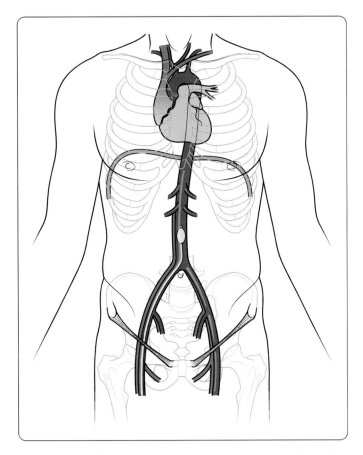

Figure 10.2 Inflation of balloon catheter in the infra-renal zone (Zone 3) to achieve pelvic inflow control.

These changes may be clinically helpful initially, but also carry a risk of potentially harmful side effects that must also be considered when choosing this method.

The principle beneficial effects include;

- Haemorrhage control
- Cardiac afterload support

As the balloon inflates, prograde perfusion below the balloon ceases due to total aortic occlusion. This leads to a near-total control of abdominal and pelvic inflow perfusion, thus reducing blood loss from the bleeding focus distal to the balloon. In addition, this aortic obstruction enhances central mean arterial pressure (MAP), thereby enhancing perfusion of organs proximal to the balloon (i.e. heart, brain). These effects may be beneficial in the arrest or peri-arrest situation where the patient has near-exsanguinated.

The magnitude to which these haemodynamic changes occur are dependent on the location of the balloon occlusion (i.e. aortic zone 1 versus zone 3). Zone 1 (i.e. descending thoracic aorta) occlusion will result in a greater reduction in arterial tree volume compared with zone 3 below the renal arteries, resulting in a higher blood pressure, as the mesenteric and renal capillary beds are not perfused. This effect can be clinically quantified by measuring systemic vascular resistance (SVR).

While it is hypothesised that this effect may be beneficial in the bleeding shocked patient, in the elective surgical context, zone 1 occlusion also incurs more profound effects on cardiac function (often mitigated in shock due to the profound hypotension already present). Roizen et al. demonstrated a reduction in ejection fraction and cardiac wall motion abnormalities on trans-oesophageal echocardiography in patients undergoing elective aortic surgery.

Furthermore, despite the advantages that REBOA can offer trauma patients in severe haemorrhagic shock, there are also potential serious deleterious physiologic side effects. The single biggest concern is REBOA-associated ischaemia-reperfusion (I-R) injury, which is a time-dependent phenomenon (length of time the balloon is inflated), where longer occlusion times are associated with a greater end-organ injury. The consequences of these effects are principally clinical, manifesting during balloon deflation, when the abdomino-pelvic viscera and extremities undergo a reintroduction of perfusion (reperfusion). A *milieu* of toxic tissue metabolites, accumulated during aortic occlusion, are delivered swiftly into both the pulmonary and systemic circulations, leading to a combination of pro-inflammatory cytokine cascade, negative inotropy and cardiac depression, profound vasodilation and pulmonary capillary dysfunction. These effects are minimised with shorter REBOA times, and current guidelines recommend keeping zone 1 and zone 3 occlusion times to under 60 and 120 minutes respectively.

Indications for REBOA use

This is still largely experimental and controversial, which is evolving as the evidence base grows. In many ways, it is easier to recognise the contra-indications to REBOA, which largely relate to the performance of older techniques, already accepted as effective in trauma (e.g. trauma thoracotomy and aortic cross-clamping), in preference over REBOA which remains investigational at this time.

Contra-indications to REBOA

- *Penetrating chest trauma with hypotension or witnessed circulatory arrest.* The gold standard of care remains a resuscitative thoracotomy where therapeutic manoeuvres (e.g. release of tamponade, control of intra-thoracic bleeding) can be performed.
- *Haemorrhage proximal to the site of the balloon.* As REBOA artificially raises central aortic pressure, bleeding from an injury proximal to this (e.g. head and neck vessels) is likely to be exacerbated with profound consequences (e.g. sudden enlargement of a neck haematoma with airway compression).

Indications for REBOA

- *Hypotension following abdominal and/or pelvic trauma.* This is the most established indication for REBOA, where the aetiology of bleeding is outside and distal to the thoracic aorta. As the patient has a preserved circulation (albeit hypotensive), the haemodynamic mechanism of REBOA is likely most effective in this setting, bridging the patient whilst awaiting definitive haemorrhage control.

- *Traumatic cardiac arrest with exsanguination.* The potential utility of REBOA in this circumstance has been described, but with very limited success at achieving a return of spontaneous circulation (ROSC). The critical window for success is more likely when a profoundly low cardiac output exists with an 'arrest' in any meaningful or survivable circulation but intrinsic myocardial contraction remains (i.e. the heart is not truly stopped). Once cardiac arrest has ensued, with loss of contractility, ROSC is doubtful (in all traumatic circumstances).
- *Anticipated cardiovascular collapse.* There may be circumstances where profound cardiovascular instability is anticipated, for example during the induction of anaesthesia or the opening of a retroperitoneal haematoma after trauma. An uninflated REBOA may be placed in the aorta in anticipation of a precipitous fall in blood pressure ready for inflation to effect temporary control as a bridge to more definitive haemostasis.

Clinical evidence

The bulk of evidence supporting the use of REBOA after trauma is currently limited to cohort studies, case series and other short reports. Quality evidence is lacking before an appropriate and widespread adoption (or discontinuation) of the technique is achievable. Several registries have been established such as Aortic Occlusion for Resuscitation in Trauma and Acute Care Surgery (AORTA) study in the United States, the Aortic Balloon Occlusion in Trauma (ABOTrauma) in Europe and the DIRECT society in Japan.

The U.S. experience has shown that REBOA is not inferior to open aortic cross-clamping *via* thoracotomy. However, overall survival was low in both groups (REBOA 28%, open clamping 16%; p = 0.12), making inferences difficult, but it was clear that REBOA could be performed expeditiously with good neurological outcomes. A small number of access site complications were reported, but without an unacceptably high incidence of procedure-related complications, supporting its feasibility.

The ABOTrauma registry described the use of REBOA either in a continuous or intermittent manner. Similar to the AORTA trial, this study also described the feasibility of implementing the technique into a treatment algorithm resulting in improved haemodynamics as a bridge to more definitive haemostasis with a moderate survival rate (43%), thereby adding further evidence of its use as an adjunct in resuscitation and haemorrhage control.

The largest studies on REBOA are from Japan, where it has been in use for more than a decade. Norii et al. performed a propensity score-matched analysis using the Japanese Trauma Databank. They demonstrated an inferior survival after blunt trauma compared the no-REBOA group with a survival odds ratio (95% confidence interval) of 0.3 (0.23–0.40); p < 0.001. However, it was felt that the application of REBOA in this circumstance was a late, last-ditch manoeuvre in severely traumatised patients where survival was poor regardless, but it did signal that harm may be associated with its use.

The current aggregate evidence base does not definitively determine whether REBOA is effective or not, which has prompted the UK-REBOA trial (a randomised Bayesian clinical trial), which compares the standard of care in torso trauma to REBOA.

Performing REBOA

A large vascular-access sheath is inserted into the common femoral artery (CFA). Using this sheath for access, a specially designed catheter is inserted under fluoroscopic guidance (radiopaque tip on balloon) and directed cephalad into position within the aortic lumen. Once at a satisfactory destination, the balloon is inflated (*via* a separate external port on the catheter) to achieve satisfactory aortic occlusion. There are five main steps:

1. Common femoral artery access
2. Sheath upsizing
3. Placement of the REBOA system
4. Balloon inflation
5. Securing the catheter

Common femoral artery access

The initial needle access may be achieved using only anatomic landmarks (i.e. pulse at the mid-inguinal point), which can be difficult to feel in the shocked patient or with ultrasound guidance (looking for arterial pulsation and direct visualisation of the needle and wire entering the vessel) (**Figure 10.3**). Percutaneous access is difficult in the moribund patient,

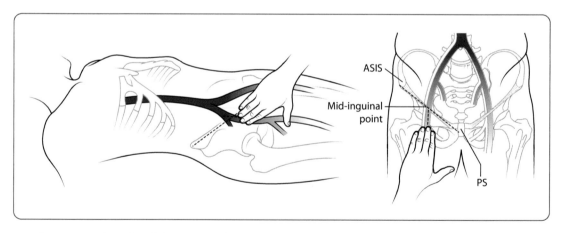

Figure 10.3 The pulse of the common femoral artery (CFA) is palpated for access. This may be difficult in the profoundly hypotensive patient, but is located anatomically at the mid-inguinal point (i.e. half way between the anterior superior iliac spine [ASIS] and the pubic symphysis [PS]). Ultrasound is a useful adjunct to visualise the vessel for direct puncture with the angioneedle.

and a cut-down may be required for direct arterial puncture. Occasionally a femoral arterial line for direct BP measurement may already be *in situ* and can be used for wire access and upgraded to fit the REBOA sheath. An angio needle is inserted percutaneously in a retrograde direction and a guidewire inserted to ensure arterial lumen access (**Figures 10.4a–f**). The needle is removed over-the-wire (OTW), while the wire is kept *in situ* and

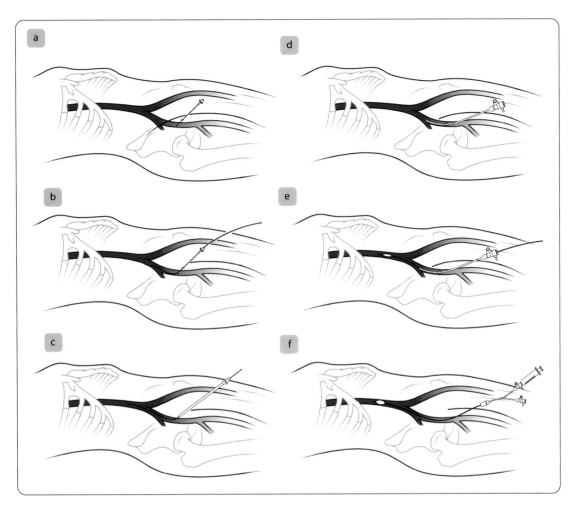

Figure 10.4 (a) Obtain common femoral artery access with an angioneedle. (b) Insert guidewire through the angioneedle. (c) Remove the angioneedle OTW (whilst keeping the wire *in situ*) and immediately follow with insertion of the sheath with dilator OTW. (d) Insert access sheath under fluoroscopic guidance. (e) Insert REBOA catheter system under fluoroscopic guidance. (f) Inflate catheter balloon.

immediately the sheath is inserted OTW and the wire subsequently removed, whilst now leaving the sheath *in situ* to act as a 'working port' for access.

Sheath upsizing

The sheath may then be exchanged OTW to the preferred size. A vessel dilator may also be used to advance arterial access. The size of the sheath required is dependent on the type of REBOA catheter in use. Once inserted, the dilator is removed OTW and the external access port of the sheath is used to confirm arterial placement (arterial pulsation) and flushed with heparinised saline.

Placement of the REBOA system

The catheter is inserted, *via* the sheath OTW (if the system requires a wire) whilst other designs use a wire-free catheter and the catheter tip directed retrograde to the aorta, ideally under fluoroscopic guidance (to minimise potential complications such as dissection, embolism, perforation or inaccurate placement). However, fluoroscopy is not always feasible or available and blind placement may be used. In addition, certain wireless REBOA catheters are licensed for fluoroscopy-free placement and distance to the required aortic zone destination is estimated by length. To improve safety around blind placement of either REBOA catheters or wires, morphometry studies have demonstrated the validity of using surface anatomic landmarks for estimating the required length of catheter and wire for safe insertion. In addition, it has been observed that there is bowing-effect of the catheter shaft during insertion due to the 'pile-driving' effect of systemic arterial pressure on the proximal aspect of the balloon. The amount of bowing is dependent upon the rigidity and strength of the catheter system. For lower-profile catheters, such as the ER-REBOA catheter, the amount of bowing is greater and the following morphometric landmarks are used for estimating insertion distance: zone 1 is the distance between the sheath insertion port to the sternal notch and zone 3 is the distance between the sheath insertion port and the xiphoid.

Balloon inflation

Using the separate external port on the catheter, the balloon is inflated to a predetermined pressure using a manual inflation device. Ideally, imaging should be obtained to confirm accurate placement of the balloon prior to inflation. In the absence of fluoroscopy, blind inflation may occur, but be aware that despite the compliant nature of the balloon, blind overinflation with aortic rupture has been reported. In addition, it is difficult to precisely know the mean aortic diameter of the patient undergoing REBOA (given the emergent nature of the procedure). However, population-based studies have estimated mean aortic size, thereby guiding the approximate inflation volume of the balloon. For example, in adults, the mean aortic diameter in zone 3 (infra-renal) is 1.3–1.9 cm and in distal zone 1 (supracoeliac) is 1.5–2.4 cm.

Ideally, additional imaging should be obtained with incremental adjustments made as required. Another surrogate marker of adequate inflation is an observed improvement in haemodynamics post-inflation. Ideally use a dilute contrast to inflate the balloon. This allows visualisation of the balloon being inflated under fluoroscopy. Diluted contrast (diluted with 0.9% saline in a ratio of 1:1 or 1:3) is used to allow easier effective balloon inflation or, more important, prevent difficulties or a delay with balloon deflation when required (due to the high viscosity of contrast agents if used without dilution).

Securing the catheter

The catheter is secured in position at a point immediately adjacent to the sheath to prevent slippage or migration pending definitive haemorrhage control, especially as the systemic arterial pressure, once augmented, will generate a substantial force on the balloon and catheter with possible migration distally if left unsecured.

Balloon deflation and device removal

Balloon deflation

Balloon deflation will result in immediate re-perfusion of the abdomino-pelvic viscera and the lower limbs that have been rendered relatively ischaemic until now (**Figure 10.5**). It is a process fraught with physiological upset and needs to be supported with appropriate

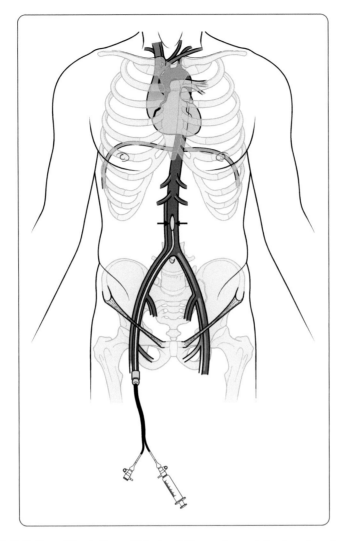

Figure 10.5 Deflation of the balloon. This should be performed slowly or in a staged manner (preferably whilst still in the operating room) to mitigate against the effects of systemic reperfusion injury and/or recurrent bleeding. Should haemodynamic collapse occur, the balloon may be immediately re-inflated.

resuscitation to mitigate the potential circulatory collapse associated with sudden systemic reperfusion. Ideally, deflation should take place in the operating (or hybrid) room, once definitive haemostasis has been achieved. However, there may be occasions where timed, partial deflation is necessary (e.g. to alleviate I-R injury or help identify bleeding sources).

Such a manoeuvre should occur after or in parallel with a well-resuscitated intravascular space, including the liberal transfusion of packed red blood cells and blood products. An active warming system should be applied to the chest and upper extremities. While the balloon is inflated, the lower extremities should not be actively warmed so as to reduce the potential I-R injury. Large metabolic derangements can occur including hyperkalaemia, calcium shifts and glucose homeostasis, and these should be actively sought and aggressively managed. A degree of hypotension is expected and is managed with fluid resuscitation, especially blood and blood products. If there is a sudden and profound drop in BP, then emergent balloon re-inflation may be necessary.

Catheter and sheath removal

Older generation REBOA systems used large-calibre sheaths (>8 Fr), requiring a formal femoral artery exposure ('arterial cut down') and subsequent repair at the termination of the procedure. Newer REBOA devices, using 7 Fr sheaths, may be removed percutaneously with manual compression, but an arterial 'cut-down' should still be considered (especially if there was difficulty with initial puncture and access, multiple puncture attempts or evidence of coagulopathy) (**Figures 10.6a,b**). The sheath should be removed as soon as possible, as a prolonged dwell time is associated with thrombosis, embolization, lower extremity ischaemia and limb loss. Anecdotally, the optimum time for sheath removal is at the conclusion of the index operation or once coagulopathy improves.

Management of REBOA-related complications

There are three broad categories of REBOA-related complications:

- Access site complications
- Deployment of the catheter and balloon complications
- Ischaemia-reperfusion injury

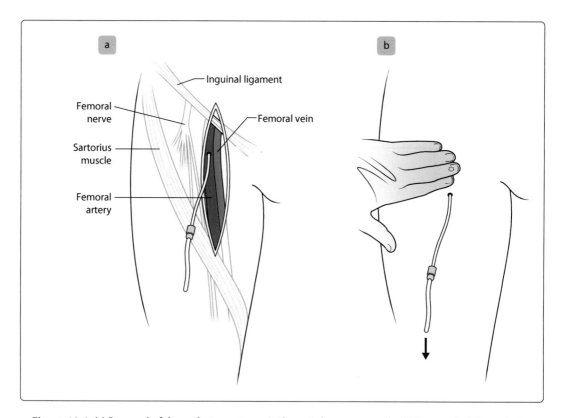

Figure 10.6 (a) Removal of the catheter system *via* the cut-down approach. (b) Removal of the catheter system percutaneously with manual compression.

Access site complications

This includes haemorrhage at the site of puncture, pseudoaneurysm formation and abscess/wound infection. Lower limb ischaemic complications have a reported incidence of 3.7%. Direct femoral arterial injury with an angioneedle can result in bleeding, either overt or even into the retroperitoneal space if a very high, posterior wall puncture occurs (incidence increases with the number of attempts at gaining vascular access and in the coagulopathic patient). Lower extremity ischaemia may occur from embolisation or direct *in situ* thrombosis of the vessel, with a reported incidence in the literature of 0.5% and an amputation rate of 0.8%. These complications appear to be directly related to sheath size, but the modern transition from larger devices to lower-profile catheters appears to have reduced this complication significantly.

Deployment of the catheter and balloon complications

Deployment of the device or advancing the balloon-catheter/wire followed by balloon inflation is generally a safe process. Potential complications include vessel wall injury (intimal flap formation, thrombosis, embolism) and vessel wall puncture (free haemorrhage or pseudoaneurysm formation). Never advance any endovascular device (wires or catheters) against resistance to avoid this problem, and ideally advance under direct fluoroscopic guidance if available or time allows. Overinflation of the balloon may also lead to aortic rupture with devastating consequences.

Ischaemia-reperfusion injury

Prolonged balloon occlusion can have a devastating effect on organ failure. Critical components to success include prompt resuscitation and timely deflation of the balloon, once definitive haemorrhage control has been achieved. Clearly, the time to balloon deflation is largely dictated by pathophysiology, rather than the surgeon, who must remain cognisant of the association of prolonged occlusion time and organ function/reperfusion injury and the potential for further haemodynamic collapse.

Future direction in the management of torso haemorrhage

In this chapter, we have focused on REBOA after torso haemorrhage, which remains a dynamic area for further research, in conjunction with other emerging technologies for haemorrhage control. As described, the biggest challenge using REBOA remains the associated I-R injury, which currently limits its use in zone 1 to 30–60 minutes. Several research avenues are being explored to ameliorate this limitation and extend the window of use. This includes the use of partial REBOA, where the balloon is partially deflated, to allow a proportion of 'flow-through' to meet the oxygen demands of tissue perfused below the balloon. This is already practiced to an extent by personnel deflating current balloon systems; however, compliant balloons in use are difficult to precisely control and the optimum flow-through has yet to be determined.

In terms of other adjuncts, several devices have been described which are going through early clinical evaluation. *Intra-abdominal foam systems* consist of a polyurethane solution, instilled into the peritoneal cavity, which then expands, providing local compression of organs and any haemorrhagic focus (i.e. akin to abdominal packing for damage control surgery). While there is a large body of compelling animal work supporting this, its use still mandates laparotomy to both explant the foam (after haemorrhage control and physiological normality is restored) and to resect any ischaemic bowel, which is known to occur with foam application (which may be dose dependent). Other areas of development include the use of *pneumatic devices* that provide direct compression to the pelvic or inguinal region. The *Abdominal Aortic and Junctional Tourniquet* is one such device, which appears to perform well in large animal models, but there is a paucity of clinical evidence surrounding its use in human patients. However, regardless of the device or modern technology used in trauma, the one overall abiding and common principle, including with old-fashioned open surgery, is that *time to effective haemorrhage control is paramount and the most important one rate-limiting step for a successful outcome.* Any future technology must also fulfil this concept!

Conflict of Interest: Dr Jonathan J. Morrison is a Clinical Advisory Board Member of Prytime Medical Inc.

Additional reading

Barnard EBG, Morrison JJ, Madureira RM et al. Resuscitative endovascular balloon occlusion of the aorta (REBOA): A population based gap analysis of trauma patients in England and Wales. *Emerg Med J* 2015;32(12):926–932.

Biffl WL, Fox CJ, Moore EE. The role of REBOA in the control of exsanguinating torso hemorrhage. *J Trauma Acute Care Surg* 2015;78(5):1054–1058.

DuBose JJ, Scalea TM, Brenner M et al. The AAST prospective Aortic Occlusion for Resuscitation in Trauma and Acute Care Surgery (AORTA) registry: Data on contemporary utilization and outcomes of aortic occlusion and resuscitative balloon occlusion of the aorta (REBOA). *J Trauma Acute Care Surg* 2016;81(3):409–419.

Gelman S, Rabbani S, Bradley ELJ. Inferior and superior vena caval blood flows during cross-clamping of the thoracic aorta in pigs. *J Thorac Cardiovasc Surg* 1988;96(3):387–392.

Jansen JO, Pallmann P, MacLennan G, Campbell MK. Bayesian clinical trial designs: Another option for trauma trials? *J Trauma Acute Care Surg* 2017;83(4):736–774.

Kamenskiy A, Miserlis D, Adamson P et al. Patient demographics and cardiovascular risk factors differentially influence geometric remodeling of the aorta compared with the peripheral arteries. *Surgery* 2015;158(6):1617–1627.

Kisat M, Morrison JJ, Hashmi ZG et al. Epidemiology and outcomes of non-compressible torso hemorrhage. *J Surg Res* 2013;184(1):414–421.

Linnebur M, Inaba K, Haltmeier T et al. Emergent non-image-guided resuscitative endovascular balloon occlusion of the aorta (REBOA) catheter placement: A cadaver-based study. *J Trauma Acute Care Surg* 2016;81(3):453–457.

MacTaggart JN, Poulson WE, Akhter M et al. Morphometric roadmaps to improve accurate device delivery for fluoroscopy-free resuscitative endovascular balloon occlusion of the aorta. *J Trauma Acute Care Surg* 2016;80(6):941–946.

Markov NP, Percival TJ, Morrison JJ et al. Physiologic tolerance of descending thoracic aortic balloon occlusion in a swine model of hemorrhagic shock. *Surgery* 2013;153(6):848–856.

Matsumura Y, Matsumoto J, Kondo H et al. Partial occlusion, conversion from thoracotomy, undelayed but shorter occlusion. *Eur J Emerg Med* 2017;1. [Epub ahead of print].

Morrison JJ. Noncompressible torso hemorrhage. *Crit Care Clin* 2017;33(1):37–54.

Morrison JJ, Galgon RE, Jansen JO et al. A systematic review of the use of resuscitative endovascular balloon occlusion of the aorta in the management of hemorrhagic shock. *J Trauma Acute Care Surg* 2015;80(2):324–334.

Morrison JJ, Percival TJ, Markov NP et al. Aortic balloon occlusion is effective in controlling pelvic hemorrhage. *J Surg Res* 2012;177(2):341–347.

Morrison JJ, Ross JD, Houston R et al. Use of resuscitative endovascular balloon occlusion of the aorta in a highly lethal model of noncompressible torso hemorrhage. *Shock* 2014;41(2):130–137.

Morrison JJ, Ross JD, Markov NP et al. The inflammatory sequelae of aortic balloon occlusion in hemorrhagic shock. *J Surg Res* 2014;191(2):423–431.

Norii T, Miyata S, Terasaka Y et al. Resuscitative endovascular balloon occlusion of the aorta in trauma patients in youth. *J Trauma Acute Care Surg* 2017;82(5):915–920.

Okada Y, Narumiya H, Ishi W, Ryoji I. Lower limb ischemia caused by resuscitative balloon occlusion of aorta. *Surg Case Reports* 2016;2(1):130.

Rago A, Duggan MJ, Marini J et al. Self-expanding foam improves survival following a lethal, exsanguinating iliac artery injury. *J Trauma Acute Care Surg* 2014;77(1):73–77.

Rago A, Marini J, Duggan M et al. Diagnosis and deployment of a self-expanding foam for abdominal exsanguination: Translational questions for human use. *J Trauma Acute Care Surg* 2015;78(3):607–613.

Rago AP, Duggan MJ, Beagle J et al. Self-expanding foam for prehospital treatment of intra-abdominal hemorrhage. *J Trauma Acute Care Surg* 2014;77:S127–S133.

Rago AP, Sharma U, Duggan M, King DR. Percutaneous damage control with self-expanding foam: Pre-hospital rescue from abdominal exsanguination. *Trauma* 2016;18(2):85–91.

Rall JM, Ross JD, Clemens MS et al. Hemodynamic effects of the Abdominal Aortic and Junctional Tourniquet in a hemorrhagic swine model. *J Surg Res* 2017;212:159–166.

Roizen MF, Beaupre PN, Alpert RA et al. Monitoring with two-dimensional transesophageal echocardiography. Comparison of myocardial function in patients undergoing supraceliac, suprarenal-infraceliac, or infrarenal aortic occlusion. *J Vasc Surg* 1984;1(2):300–305.

Russo RM, Neff LP, Lamb CM et al. Partial resuscitative endovascular balloon occlusion of the aorta in swine model of hemorrhagic shock. *J Am Coll Surg* 2016;223(2):359–368.

Sadeghi M, Nilsson KF, Larzon T et al. The use of aortic balloon occlusion in traumatic shock: First report from the ABO trauma registry. *Eur J Trauma Emerg Surg* 2017;(123456789):1–11.

Søvik E, Stokkeland P, Storm BS et al. The use of aortic occlusion balloon catheter without fluoroscopy for life-threatening post-partum haemorrhage. *Acta Anaesthesiol Scand* 2012;56(3):388–393.

Stokland O, Miller M, Ilebekk A, Kiil F. Mechanism of hemodynamic responses to occlusion of the descending thoracic aorta. *Am J Physiol Hear Circ Physiol* 1980;238:H423–H429.

Teeter W, Matsumoto J, Idoguchi K et al. Smaller introducer sheaths for REBOA may be associated with fewer complications. *J Trauma Acute Care Surg* 2016;81(6):1039–1045.

Index